Everybody's Guide to Chiropractic Health Care

Also by the author:

The Palmistry Workbook
The Nonviolent Revolution
Lovelight: Unveiling the Mysteries of Sex and
  Romance (with Julia Bondi)
Living with Asthma

EVERYBODY'S GUIDE TO CHIROPRACTIC HEALTH CARE

Nathaniel Altman

Foreword by Fred H. Barge, D.C., Ph.C.
President, International Chiropractors Association

JEREMY P. TARCHER, INC.
Los Angeles

This book is dedicated to

Adelson de Barros

Library of Congress Cataloging in Publication Data

Altman, Nathaniel, 1948–
    Everybody's guide to chiropractic health care / Nathaniel Altman;
foreword by Fredrick H. E. Barge.
        p.   cm.
    Includes bibliographical references.
    1. Chiropractic.   2. Health.   I. Title.
    RZ241.A48   1990
    615.5'34—dc20   89-48641
    ISBN 0-87477-560-4   CIP

Jeremy P. Tarcher, Inc.
5858 Wilshire Blvd., Suite 200
Los Angeles, CA 90036

Distributed by St. Martin's Press, New York

Manufactured in the United States of America
10 9 8 7 6 5 4 3 2

Contents

Acknowledgments

I would like to express my thanks to the following people whose varied contributions were essential to the successful completion of the manuscript: Fred H. Barge, D.C., Ph.C., for his foreword, and for sharing his expertise in chiropractic philosophy and practice; Frank Wilheit, D.C., of Palmer College of Chiropractic for his information about adjustment techniques; Martha Painter of Sherman College of Straight Chiropractic for her helpful suggestions and chiropractic literature; Todd Herold, D.C., for the photos of him giving chiropractic adjustments to children; and William N. Borkon of the Pennsylvania College of Straight Chiropractic for giving me the run of the library. I am especially grateful to Jackie Knowles, D.C., and Donald Epstein, D.C., for reviewing the manuscript, as well as for their encouragement, support, and helpful suggestions.

I would also like to gratefully acknowledge help and/or permission from the following corporations: the Foundation of Chiropractic Education and Research for permission to reproduce several anatomical drawings from *Chiropractic Health Care*; the International Chiropractors Association, the American Chiropractic Association, and the Federation of Straight Chiropractic Organizations for generously supplying me a wealth of reference material; the Wellcome Trustees for the graphic depicting early spinal manipulation and traction; Ebury Press for the graphic of the spinal column; Eleanor Gilpatrick for her charts concerning attitudes toward health and nutrition; Dr. Bertram Spector for his graphics concerning Moiré contourography; Murdoch

Engineering, Inc., for their photograph of the thermeter; Williams Manufacturing for the photograph of their Zenith® Hylo™ adjusting table; Canadian Memorial Chiropractic College for the photos of D. D. Palmer and B. J. Palmer; Palmer College of Chiropractic and Cleveland Chiropractic College (Kansas City) for their photos depicting adjusting techniques; and the Parker Chiropractic Research Foundation for their chart on the effects of spinal misalignments.

Foreword

Someone once observed that if we waited for a book that absolutely agrees with everyone's opinion on a subject, then no books would ever be printed. Certainly this is a true observation, and as I read *Everybody's Guide to Chiropractic Health Care*, those thoughts ran through my mind. I am sure that if a layman wrote a text entitled *Medicine Today*, the medical profession would find among its many authorities both those who extolled and those who condemned the book. This book, too, will have those chiropractors who will wish that it presented only their particular chiropractic viewpoint. But *Chiropractic Health Care* was not written for chiropractors; it was written for health-care consumers searching for an alternative to ordinary medical care, and in this perspective it does a superlative job.

I have practiced chiropractic for thirty-five years. I was the ninth in my family to pursue this profession; our family of chiropractors now numbers fifteen. Two of my daughters became D.C.'s, one a C.T., and I have three chiropractor sons-in-law. I have been a fortunate man to travel the world of chiropractic in my writing, teaching, and lecturing vocations. I say this not to establish my authority, but rather to lend credibility to my endorsement of this text.

I personally believe that no other book today explains so well the many complexities and forms of practice of this emerging profession. At this writing, chiropractic approaches its one hundredth year of existence. It is not an infant profession; I would place it in its most difficult adolescent years. Finally throwing off the chains placed upon it by organized medicine but still struggling for its identity, chiropractic now faces its era of responsibility, its age of maturity.

The profession must spell out once and for all its major tenets, its definition, scope of practice, and standards of practice and care. Within the framework of how chiropractic presents itself today, Nathaniel Altman has truly accomplished a remarkable task. This book explains in a congenial and knowledgeable way the differences of thought that separate the practice of "mixer" and "straight" chiropractic. The liberal "mixer" concepts are not demeaned but placed in the context of what is useful for you, the patient, the consumer of health services. The conservative "straight" concepts are explained in the light of what always has been taught in chiropractic.

Chiropractic teaches that the body is a self-healing organism and that the chiropractor's role is to restore proper spinal alignment through vertebral adjustment, thus freeing the body of nerve interference caused by spinal subluxations (or misalignments). The body free of nerve interference between the central nervous system and its organs, bones, tissues, and muscles then performs its own healing miracles.

Altman clearly explains that chiropractic does not hold out a cure or a treatment for disease. Chiropractors simply adjust the spine to free the body of nerve interference. This allows the body to affect its own cure, so to speak. Chiropractic recognizes that the true cause of disease lies within. When the body is functioning properly it can adequately comprehend its environment; when it is not, then external factors such as germs, viruses, allergens, insects, and carcinogenic chemicals can raise havoc and create what we call disease.

Contemporary medical author Dennis T. Jaffe, Ph.D., makes a similar observation in his book *Healing From Within*:

"Of course, disease-producing microorganisms are always present, but usually they can be fought off successfully. However, some individuals never get sick, while others pick up every cold in the neighborhood. So although the germ may be one of the essential and contributing causes, it alone is not sufficient to produce illness."

I agree. *External* factors alone are not sufficient to produce illness. First the individual must be susceptible to the problem. Because *internal* factors determine the nature of our reaction to outside agents of disease, the true cause of disease lies within the body itself. This fact is one of the major tenets of chiropractic philosophy and is the cornerstone of the unique philosophical approach that chiropractic provides for patient care and the maintenance of health.

Medical authors today widely agree with chiropractic's "cause from within" concepts. Dr. Andrew Weil, M.D., states in his popular book *Health and Healing* that "the true causes of disease are internal." He goes on to say: "This principle suggests other ways of thinking about prevention and treatment than those predominant in conventional medicine. Rather than warring on disease agents with the hope (vain, I suspect) of eliminating them, we ought to worry more about strengthening resistance to them and learning to live in balance with them more of the time."

Dr. D. D. Palmer, the founder of chiropractic, made a similar statement in 1910 in *The Science, Art and Philosophy of Chiropractic*: "The science of chiropractic has modified our views concerning life, death, health, and disease. We no longer believe that disease is an entity, something foreign to the body, which may enter from without, and with which we have to grasp, struggle, fight and conquer, or submit and succumb to its ravages. Disease is a disturbed condition, not a thing of enmity. Disease is an abnormal performance of certain functions; the abnormal activity has its causes."

As Dr. Palmer stated, "abnormal activity has its causes." Chiropractic science has found that this "cause from within" is often a misalignment in the spine called *subluxation*. This malposition of the spinal vertebrae causes nerve interference that can produce malfunction. The malfunction in turn causes lowered tissue resistance, faulty body coordination between its many systems, and resulting disease. As the cause is within, so too the cure lies within. If we improve the body's ability to function properly, it will throw off, and ward off, disease. And to ward off disease should be our greatest concern rather than trying to patch up the damage later on. As Dr. Robert A. Aldrich, M.D., Professor of Preventive Medicine, University of Colorado, states: "The maintenance of health should take precedence over the treatment of disease." With this statement, chiropractors heartily concur.

So, with this brief introduction I will now turn the reader over to this book. Nathaniel Altman does a masterful job of explaining the many differing modes of chiropractic philosophy and practice. For you, the health-care consumer and patient, this work will be a welcome guide to chiropractic understanding. With the public understanding of what chiropractic is will come an awareness of the roles of self and body in the cause and cure of disease. This awareness will stop the foolish and costly war against germs and agents of disease. People will look to themselves for the causes of their problems. From their increased awareness of the true causes of disease will come a physical moral code that will go a long way in our quest for true health.

May Dr. D. D. Palmer's prediction come true: *"In the near future chiropractic will be as much valued for its preventative qualities as it now is for adjusting and relieving the cause of ailments."*

Enjoy this book. After you better understand the chiropractic profession, may you also enjoy the comprehensive health benefits of chiropractic care.

Fred H. Barge, D.C., Ph.C.
President, International Chiropractors Association

The Chiropractic Alternative

During the past two decades, America has witnessed a ground swell of interest in alternative forms of health care. There is every indication that this trend will continue to the end of the century and beyond. *Chiropractic* is one of those alternative ways to health, and in less than one hundred years it has become the largest drugless health system in the Western world. Developed in the United States by Daniel David Palmer in 1895, chiropractic is now the second largest health-care system in North America, after conventional (*allopathic*) medicine. Despite many years of desperate attempts by the American Medical Association and other groups to suppress its growth, more than 13 million Americans choose chiropractic every year.

Chiropractic is a unique health-care science that deals with the vital relationship between the nervous system and the spinal column, and with the role of this relationship in the restoration and maintenance of health. The philosophy of chiropractic teaches that our ability to adapt to changes in our bodies and our environment is essential to the maintenance of life and health. It also teaches that an unobstructed flow of mental impulses from the brain through the spinal nerves and onward to every body cell will help us achieve the balance, harmony, and vitality we need to enjoy vibrant health and a long, productive life.

The major premise of chiropractic states that vertebrae of the spine can, and frequently do, become misaligned, causing interference to the normal conduction of nerve impulses from the brain to the organs and tissues of the body. Although most spinal misalignments are corrected naturally through normal body movement, some become fixated. As a result, normal nerve transmission is impaired for long periods of time and our health suffers.

What distinguishes doctors of chiropractic (or D.C.'s) from other health professionals is that they work primarily to identify, analyze, and adjust these vertebrae (and related structures such as the pelvis) back to their correct positions. When vertebral misalignments are corrected, chiropractors believe that a major limitation to the body's health potential is eliminated. Consequently, our ability to experience a state of health is enhanced.

Contrary to popular belief, the scope of chiropractic extends far beyond the treatment of back pains and stiff necks. Although symptoms of back and neck pain do respond favorably to chiropractic care, chiropractic is recognized for its ability to promote the total health and integration of the body—it focuses on the ability of the body to heal itself *from the inside out.* Chiropractic encourages us to take personal responsibility for our lives by teaching us to preserve our health rather than merely treating the symptoms of disease. It is in harmony with such modern trends as healthy eating, exercise, and holistic health care.

The cost of chiropractic care is roughly half that of conventional medical therapy. This effective and economical way to cope with America's health crisis offers great promise to those who suffer from ill health as well as to those who want to stay healthy and active throughout their lives. Chiropractic cannot guarantee a state of positive wellness—no health-care system can. However, the primary goal of chiropractic is to help lay the foundation for positive wellness by keeping the nervous system free from the impingements caused by misalignment of the spine and related structures.

Since its beginning, chiropractic has helped millions of people around the world achieve their potential for positive wellness. They have found that the preventive approach of chiropractic has helped keep them healthy at reasonable cost. Chiropractic adjustments, greatly refined since 1895, have relieved their painful back and neck problems including whiplash injuries, neuralgia, sciatica, bursitis, tendonitis, lumbago, disc problems, and muscle sprains. In addition, chiropractic has been successful in helping their bodies control organic disorders such as hypertension, arthritis, chronic fatigue, heart trouble, and a host of other ailments, some of which did not respond well to medical therapy.

Chiropractic patients come from all backgrounds, encompassing preschool children, retired adults, Olympic athletes, factory workers, professional dancers, secretaries, teachers, farmers, mail carriers, truck drivers, firefighters, homemakers, and architects. A wide spectrum of outstanding Americans—among them Harry S Truman, Eleanor Roosevelt, Hubert Humphrey, Jimmy Connors, John McEnroe, Tracy Austin, Bruce Jenner, Melvin Belli, Burt Reynolds, and Rocky Marciano—have been among chiropractic's enthusiastic supporters.

This book will introduce you to the science and art of chiropractic and how it can help keep you well. Part One explains what chiropractic is and how it works with your body's natural ability to heal itself from the inside out. In Part Two, you will learn what it can do for you, how long it takes to get well, and what happens when you visit a chiropractor. This part also focuses on the chiropractic profession itself and explores modern chiropractic education and professional standards, to help you select your personal chiropractor. Part Three explores what chiropractors call "constructive survival values," offering practical guidance regarding stress management, diet, and exercise which you can follow to prevent spinal misalignments and to enhance the benefits of regular chiropractic care.

Whether you are currently enjoying good health and want to optimize it, or are bothered by a problem that does not respond to conventional medical therapy, chiropractic is worth looking into. This book will help you make an informed decision about the value of chiropractic care and will show you how to fight the high cost of health care today.

PART ONE

*Seeking Wellness:
The Foundations
of Chiropractic*

CHAPTER 1

The Promise of Chiropractic

A middle-aged executive nearly gave up his job because his migraine headaches were, as he said, "driving me up the wall." After six chiropractic adjustments, both the frequency and intensity of his headaches were sharply reduced.

A young woman had not had her period in three years. After four months of chiropractic care, she resumed her normal menstrual cycle.

A handyman sprained his back lifting machinery and could barely walk. Five minutes after a chiropractic adjustment, he was playfully lifting the chiropractor's child and tossing him into the air.

A teenage girl was taking six prescription drugs to control nine different allergies. After three weeks of chiropractic care, she was free of allergy symptoms and stopped taking drugs.

A fifty-year-old man was told that he needed surgery to repair a herniated disc. After only two chiropractic adjustments, he returned to his amazed physician, who canceled the operation.

An elderly woman dying of cancer received regular chiropractic care in place of narcotic drugs. Although she did not have a remission, she was able to live her last days with dignity.

If you walk into any chiropractor's office, the chances are good that patients like these will eagerly relate the "miracles" they have experienced thanks to chiropractic: "Chiropractic cured my back trouble." "It gave me sleep after years of insomnia and sleeping pills." "It helped lower my blood pressure." "My arthritis is finally under control." "My child is no longer hyperactive and is doing better in school." "Chiropractic has relieved my constipation."

Before reviewing the evidence from nearly a century of clinical research, it is important to know that chiropractic was designed primarily not to treat symptoms but to help the body restore optimum nerve function. Chiropractic maintains that disturbances to the nervous system, such as *subluxations* (a condition in which one or more *vertebrae* are out of alignment to the extent that a nerve is impinged and normal transmission of nerve energy is obstructed), can be the cause of aggravated *dis-ease* (disorder within the body, from the original derivation of *disease* meaning "lack of ease"), which may eventually lead to disease symptoms. As a result of reflex action, almost any part of the nervous system may directly or indirectly cause symptomatic reactions in another part of the body. For example, a subluxation of the third cervical vertebra, located in the neck area, may trigger a headache, an asthmatic syndrome, or another nerve-related problem, although it may not be the sole cause.

Since every tissue and organ of the body is connected to and controlled by nerves from the spinal cord and brain, removal of nerve interference can bring dramatic results. With careful adjustments (see Figure 1–1), the chiropractor releases our natural healing forces, which have the potential to relieve almost every ailment known, including heart disease, asthma, and cancer.

Here we must differentiate between two chiropractic terms, *adjustments* and *manipulation*. The vast majority of chiropractic adjustments involve the application of a sudden and precise force (known in the profession as a "dynamic thrust") to a specific point of the vertebra *with the primary intention of allowing the body to remove nerve interfer-*

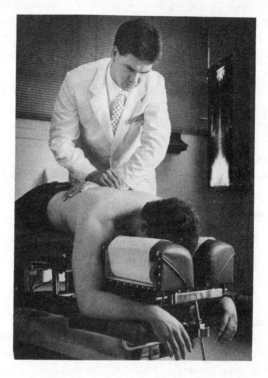

Figure 1–1. A chiropractor administering an adjustment to the thoracic area of the spine. (Photo courtesy of Cleveland Chiropractic College, Kansas City)

ence. It is the body's reaction to the applied force that realigns structure as a secondary effect. However, some procedures, such as the sacro-occipital technique, or SOT, are light-touch reflex adjustments that can also remove nerve interference. A manipulation, in contrast, is often a nonspecific, generalized procedure that mobilizes joints, increases range of movement, or realigns joint structure with the intent to stimulate or inhibit body functions. For example, a practitioner who massages and then twists the neck and head in order to bring about a greater range of movement would be performing a manipulation.

Some chiropractors claim that because an adjustment is far more precise than a manipulation, it is often more effective in removing nerve interference. In addition, they point out that as chiropractors they receive more extensive and specialized training in spinal anatomy, biomechanics, and structural disturbances and their correction than any other health professional. Though much of the following evidence is based on manipulation, which is often performed by osteopaths and physical therapists, positive results can be equaled and commonly surpassed by specific chiropractic adjustments.

The Scope of Chiropractic

Most people think that chiropractors work only with orthopedic (musculoskeletal) cases, such as backache, whiplash, disc pain, and sciatica. Although the majority of patients come to chiropractors with musculoskeletal complaints, many go to chiropractors for other functional disorders that involve major body organs and processes. According to Dr. Chester A. Wilk, a chiropractor who spearheaded a successful antitrust suit against the American Medical Association in 1976, the following ailments have responded favorably to chiropractic care:

Type M: Musculoskeletal Disorders

lumbar (lower back) strain or sprain	arthritic conditions
	sciatica
cervical (neck) syndromes	sprains
dorsal (midback) conditions	spinal distortion
	torticollis (wryneck)
cerebrospinal disorders	sacroiliac strains
whiplash injuries	bursitis

Type O: Organic Conditions

headache
nervous disorders
common cold
neuritis
neurological disease
high blood pressure
respiratory conditions

gastrointestinal disorders
sinusitis
migraine
bronchial asthma
emotional problems
heart trouble

This list of ailments is impressive, but chiropractic should not be viewed as a cure-all for every one of these disorders. First, there are other factors in addition to nerve interference that influence ill health. These include poor diet, overwork, poor adaptation to stress, environmental pollution, heredity, alcohol and drug abuse, and even a possible subconscious intention to be sick. Second, some conditions respond better to chiropractic care than others do. They depend, in part, on the individual's basic constitution, the length of illness, and the severity of the patient's condition.

Chiropractors such as Dr. Carl Tompkins, who has thirty years' experience caring for thousands of patients, remind us that disease symptoms are often the final stage of a long process of dis-ease. Many people consult a chiropractor as a last resort after medical science has failed them. Although chiropractic care has helped millions of people recover from chronic health problems, it does not offer miracle cures. For this reason, a good chiropractor will make no promises. He or she may tell you that people who manifest a condition such as yours have responded favorably to chiropractic care in the past, or that the removal of nerve interference may in turn help your body to overcome a health problem.

Since the days of the founder, Daniel David Palmer, chiropractic has been exiled to the fringes of the health-care mainstream by the organized medical profession. As a result, chiropractic has been denied the private and public funding that has gone toward medical research. Most of the data concerning the effectiveness of chiropractic has therefore been collected by chiropractors themselves. Yet, even as organized medicine condemns it, conventional medical research also offers an abundance of data that directly and indirectly attests to the value of chiropractic as a safe, effective means to help patients overcome a wide variety of ailments.

Relief for Musculoskeletal Disorders

The most common complaints among chiropractic patients may be sore backs, stiff necks, and disc problems, but arthritis, rheumatism, sciatica, gout, postural deformities, muscle spasm, whiplash, nerve conditions, and tennis elbow and other kinds of sports injuries are also problems that lead people to seek chiropractic care.

An article from the British Medical Journal in 1955, titled "Low Back Pain Treated by Manipulation," reported that 50 percent of the patients treated by spinal manipulation were free of symptoms by the end of one week. Only 27 percent of those receiving bed rest and drugs could claim similar results. Within three weeks, 87 percent of the manipulated patients were discharged from treatment, whereas only 60 percent of the others were.

A 1977 study of records from the Wisconsin Worker's Compensation Fund compared chiropractic with medical care in cases of industrial back injuries. The average compensation time for a chiropractic patient was 13.2 days at a cost of $145.64 (in 1977 dollars). A patient receiving medical care was compensated 18.3 days at an average cost of $267.58. Similar results were reported in occupational back injury studies in California in 1970, Montana in 1978, and at the University of Wisconsin in 1979. The following year, researchers in Oregon found chiropractic care to offer a 57 percent savings over medical care in the treatment of industrial back injuries.

In 1988, a study involving the Florida Department of Labor and Employment Security completed a comprehensive analysis of claims for back-related injuries. Based on a total of 52,091 injuries, it was found that chiropractic patients had the lowest incidence of compensation injuries when compared to medical or osteopathic patients. In addition, of the patients who had compensable injuries, chiropractic patients were less likely to undergo hospitalization. Finally, chiropractic care cost nearly half the cost of medical therapy: $558 as compared to $1100.

Foreign studies also have yielded positive results. According to the German journal *Manuelle Medezin*, in a study of 43 patients who had suffered traumatic injury to the spine, after only 1 chiropractic adjustment 51.8 percent were symptom free. In another German study of 106 patients with cranial trauma, two-thirds were symptom free after an average of 2.8 chiropractic adjustments. At the University of Saskatchewan Hospital in Canada, 287 patients with low back pain were given daily spinal adjustments for one to three weeks. The results of this study, published in the March 1985 issue of *The Canadian Family Physician*, reported that 71 percent of all patients with low back pain returned to normal or near-normal ability, and 87 percent of all patients with posterior joint and/or sacro-iliac joint syndrome returned to normal or near normal after the series of chiropractic adjustments. Other medical studies have related rheumatoid arthritis to compression of the spinal nerves by bones. Sciatica, neuralgia, lumbago, and intercostal neuritis also have been linked to misalignments of the spine.

Another common disorder caused by spinal nerve compression is *referred pain*, which is pain perceived by the brain as coming from a site other than its true origin. As early as 1933, research by Neville T. Ussher, M.D., found that spinal curvature resulting in nerve interference could produce radiating pain in different parts of the body with symptoms resembling gall bladder disease, appendicitis, gastritis, ulcer, colitis, spastic constipation, and other forms of irritation. The *Journal of the American Medical Association* reported in 1971 that a ruptured vertebral disc could produce a pain that simulates angina. In January 1948, the *American Heart Journal* reported that nerve root pain in the midback can simulate, and is often mistaken for, coronary heart disease. As in a heart attack, the pain can radiate to the jaw or the upper left arm and even cause a choking sensation in the throat. In some cases, spinal manipulation brought immediate relief.

The fact that chiropractic can correct the cause of many musculoskeletal disorders was emphasized by the prestigious Commission of Inquiry into Chiropractic in New Zealand. It undertook the most complete and objective study of the science to date. Authorized by the governor-general, the commission heard testimony from hundreds of chiropractors and their patients, medical doctors, physiotherapists, and independent researchers from around the world. In its report, presented to the New Zealand Parliament in 1979, the commission stated: "There can be no doubt that chiropractic treatment is effective for musculoskeletal spinal disorders. As well as back pain, which makes up the great bulk of chiropractic practice, these must be taken to include migraine and pain radiating from the spine."

Chiropractic and Organic Disorders

All major organs of the body are closely linked to the nervous system radiating from the spine. The wide variety of visceral disorders (involving the internal organs) that occur when spinal subluxations cause nerve interference should come as no surprise. Nevertheless, the list is impressive. Let's start with the head and move down.

The seven cervical vertebrae (those that make up the neck) can become subluxated by excessive physical, chemical, or emotional stress. Such misalignments can irritate the nerve roots in the neck, which can, in turn, cause minor constriction in some of the blood vessels to the brain, producing headache. The New Zealand report included results of a study of 87 migraine headache victims who received chiropractic adjustments over a two-year period. Some 78 percent of the females and 75 percent of the males suffering from "classical migraine" reported marked improvement.

An Australian study of migraine headache at the University of New South Wales compared chiropractic adjustments with manipulation by medical doctors and physiotherapists. Results showed that after two months, the chiropractic group experienced a 40 percent reduction in frequency of attack and a 43 percent reduction in pain intensity. The others reported only 34 percent reduction in frequency of attack and the same reduction in pain intensity. The findings confirmed the results of an earlier study in Germany that attributed 80 percent of all headaches to vertebral subluxations. A 1969 study featured in *The Canadian Family Physician* found that "at least 70 percent" of head pain arises from problems of the cervical spine and related structures.

Other research has shown that whiplash injury can damage nerves affecting the ear, as well as cause recurring dizziness. Excessive motion of a cervical vertebra also caused dizziness and blurred vision. A letter published in the British medical journal *Lancet* linked vertigo to subluxations in the neck. Irritation of the cervical nerves was related to nausea, headache, transitory deafness, blurred vision, and loss of balance. The 1970 *Yearbook of the Academy of Applied Osteopathy* included a series of manipulative techniques for the treatment of eye conditions such as retinitis, conjunctivitis, early cataract, and glaucoma. And the *Journal of the American Osteopathic Association* discovered that 88 percent of subjects with cervical lesions (subluxations) also suffered from thyroid dysfunctions, compared with

34 percent of thyroid dysfunction among subjects without cervical disturbance.

The *Annals of Allergy* explained that spinal curvature, which is correctable by manipulation, may interfere with the central nervous system and aggravate asthma. The *Journal of the American Osteopathic Association* discussed the beneficial uses of manipulation for the midback as an adjunct to diet and breathing exercises for asthmatics. Other medical references have drawn attention to the ability of spinal manipulation to lower blood pressure, fight against chronic lung disease, and improve the body's use of oxygen.

An article in a European medical journal described a case study on 100 ulcer patients and found that 86 percent suffered from spinal curvatures of some kind and 90 percent showed pathological changes in the intervertebral discs. A 1967 report by the renowned Mayo Clinic related both urinary retention and incontinence to misaligned discs in the lower back.

Problems related to the sex organs also have been linked to spinal misalignments. The German journal *Manuelle Medezin* presented several arguments in favor of spinal manipulation for a variety of female disorders before and after giving birth. An article in the *Archives of Physical Medicine and Rehabilitation* and a letter in the *Journal of the American Medical Association* explained the physiological relationship between male sexual dysfunction and misalignments in the lower back.

Cancer.   John has cancer, but after four months of chiropractic care he is in remission. Does this mean that chiropractic cures cancer? A responsible chiropractor would answer in the negative, but proceed to ask a more important question: Can a physiologically sound organism, freed from nerve interference, fight cancer? The answer to *this* question is yes. Early evidence that vertebral subluxations could be directly linked to decreased immunologic competence in human beings was presented by the Soviet physician A. D. Speransky in 1944. This was later reaffirmed in E. D. Gardner's *Fundamentals of Neurology*, which said that autonomic functions of the nervous system (such as resistance to disease) are affected by spinal trauma. When nerve interference is removed, normal neural activity can return.

Years ago, physicians believed that glands alone governed the immune system. However, present medical thought holds that the nerves play an important role in the body's immune response. Research has linked the nervous system to immunity by way of its control of glandular functions. The thymus gland, considered of vital importance in immune response, has been shown to be directly influenced by central nervous system activity. According to Blair Justice, Ph.D., of the University of Texas Health Science Center in Houston, "The brain, nervous system, immune system, and endocrine system may be so closely linked that they constitute a single regulatory network in the body."

These findings are of value both in the prevention and treatment of cancer. To the degree that the nervous system is functioning at an optimal level, the greater the body's ability to resist harmful bacteria and viruses, including cancer cells. An article in the March 13, 1973, issue of *Time* magazine included the following comments regarding this important issue:

Sir Frank MacFarlane Burnet, an Australian, and Dr. Lewis Thomas, who has just been appointed President of Memorial Sloane-Kettering Cancer Center, suggested a relationship between the immune system and cancerous growth. They postulated that in addition to protecting the body from invaders, the immune system has the duty to police cell growth and prevent the survival and reproduction of abnormal or "outlaw" cells.

William Burrow's *Textbook of Microbiology* agrees: "Cases of spontaneous regression of human tumors suggest that an active immunological response may be holding the growth in check."

Responsible chiropractors will never promise that they can cure cancer, although Dr. Tedd Koren, a chiropractor, believes that chiropractic is beneficial whether or not the patient is under the care of a medical doctor. In the *International Review of Chiropractic*, Koren pointed out that cancer is the result of a body not working correctly for many years. Removing nerve interference by chiropractic adjustments may help a body that works improperly to work properly. In effect, it has a better chance of fighting off cancer. For those under medical care, Dr. Koren feels an uninterrupted nerve supply will help increase the patient's natural resistance, thereby lessening the chances of *iatrogenic disease*, or disease induced as a consequence of medical therapy (such as radiation).

AIDS. Many of these comments about cancer also can be applicable to a disease such as AIDS. Since the beginning of the AIDS epidemic in 1980, chiropractic has been recognized by patients and practitioners as a valuable adjunct to both medical and alternative therapies. According to the book *Psychoimmunity and the Healing Process*, edited by Jason Serinus: "Chiropractic alignment of the body, specifically to alleviate stress and tensions placed on the medulla oblongata and the coccyx, is important in cases of AIDS and immune dysfunction." Chiropractic adjustments are recommended to open up neurological pathways to help restore the proper functioning of nervous and endocrine systems of the body.

Tom O'Connor, who was diagnosed with ARC (AIDS-related complex), pursued alternative methods to avoid coming down with the opportunistic infections and body lesions that occur when ARC becomes AIDS. After six years, not only did he not come down with AIDS but his health improved. Part of his program included chiropractic, especially the sacro-occipital technique, known as SOT (described in chapter 7). In his book *Living with AIDS*, O'Connor spoke highly of chiropractic care: "I derive great benefit from these visits. Chiropractic has enhanced my sense of responsibility for my body's health." He concluded, "A visit to a competent chiropractor should benefit anyone, especially those whose immune system cannot afford to be further impaired by a structural nervous dysfunction."

Chiropractic Findings

In the previous pages we reviewed a small part of the extensive medical literature concerning ailments that respond to spinal manipulation and chiropractic adjustments. Although some critics feel that chiropractic literature is less objective than data from other sources, the following may help us understand why so many people feel chiropractic has brought hope when medical science was unable to help them.

A partial listing of cases successfully treated at Spears Chiropractic Hospital in Denver (the only chiropractic inpatient facility in the world) includes incapacitating headaches, triple vision and blackouts, convulsions, disability due to stroke, rheumatoid arthritis, cerebral palsy, muscular dystrophy, hyperthyroidism, goiter, emphysema, bronchitis, and several skin disorders including scleroderma (thickening of the skin) and vascular dermatitis. Many of these ailments had been previously diagnosed by medical doctors.

Lyle W. Sherman, D.C., saw dramatic results while he was head of the Palmer Chiropractic Clinic in Davenport, Iowa. According to Sherman, some of the ailments that responded to chiropractic care included cirrhosis and cancer of the liver, epilepsy, encephalitis, hydrocephalus, tumors, and multiple sclerosis.

The most impressive reports on chiropractic's success with paralysis were published in *The Chiropractic Story* by Marcus Bach, Ph.D. Winifred Gardella, the 1955 March of Dimes poster girl, underwent two-and-a-half years of unsuccessful medical treatment to restore her lifeless arms and legs. A chiropractor heard of her case, and after six months of chiropractic adjustments she put her crutches aside and walked. Another dramatic case involved eleven-year-old Donny Spackman of suburban Chicago. Confined to a wheelchair with paralysis, after ten days of chiropractic care he got out of his wheelchair and walked.

Chiropractic's effect on blood pressure also has been documented. Dr. R. P. Hood, a Kansas chiropractor, studied 60 patients with hypertension. In addition to diet therapy and a regular exercise program, Dr. Hood gave each patient an average of 9.8 chiropractic adjustments over a period of 71 days. By the end of the study, the average systolic blood pressure fell from 163 mm Hg to 130.4 mm Hg, and the average diastolic pressure fell to 82 mm Hg from 93.8 mm Hg. His investigations also included 8 patients with low blood pressure, who received an average of 5.5 adjustments over 72.4 days. By the end of the program, their average systolic blood pressure went up from 100 mm Hg to 114 mm Hg, and the diastolic rose to 76.3 mm Hg from 67.5 mm Hg. Writing in the *Digest of Chiropractic Economics*, Dr. Hood claimed: "Evidence is overwhelming that abnormal blood pressures either rise or fall toward the optimum as vertebral subluxations are reduced." A less ambitious study reported by the Foundation of Chiropractic Education and Research did not include diet and exercise, but merely the correction of vertebral subluxations. In this investigation of patients with hypertension, an average 10–20 mm Hg drop in blood pressure was reported.

Although the New Zealand Commission of Inquiry into Chiropractic heard many cases similar to these, it was unable to conclude that chiropractic would guarantee such positive results all the time. After reviewing hundreds of cases, the commission prepared the following carefully worded statement:

> On the question whether spinal manual therapy [chiropractic adjustments] can influence organic and/or visceral disorders, the Commission is satisfied that in some cases this is at least a possibility. Moreover, there is enough anecdotal material to satisfy the Commission that in some instances chiropractors have been able to relieve disorders of this nature which seem to have defeated orthodox medicine. . . . Without [the chiropractor], the quality of life of many would be less bearable. Their pain and frustration are undoubtedly relieved.

Psychological Well-Being

It is well known that a healthy nervous system is basic to good mental health. Nerve impairments can produce localized stress or psychological syndromes such as depression or hyperactivity. A study of delinquent children undertaken at Yale University found that 98.6 percent of the more violent youths had at least one sign of neurological impairment, as opposed to 66.7 percent of the less violent group.

Although extensive comparative studies still need to be done, several pilot studies have indicated that regular chiropractic care can have a dramatic effect on people with severe emotional problems. The first pilot study was performed by G. W. Hartmann, Ph.D., and Herman Schwartz,

D.C. Sponsored by the National Committee on Psychology of the American Chiropractic Association in 1947, it involved 350 children and adults, 114 of whom were institutionalized. All the patients were evaluated before the testing began. Seventy-five percent of those who had undergone medical and psychiatric therapy showed no change in their progress. Only 13 percent reported some improvement. Ten percent (or 35) reported that their progress had deteriorated.

After receiving regular chiropractic adjustments, an impressive 81 percent of the patients were found to have experienced a marked improvement. Four percent (or 13) of the participants showed no improvement. Only 6 patients (1.5 percent of the total) were found to be worse than before treatment started. Approximately 42 percent of the patients received no psychotherapy while under chiropractic care, and only 8.5 percent received in-depth psychiatric counseling during the course of the investigation.

A more recent study by the Psychoeducational and Guidance Services in Texas compared conventional methods of treatment with chiropractic. It was carried out during the school year of 1973–1974 with 24 children who showed marked behavioral and learning problems due to neurological dysfunction. By the end of the study, the results showed that spinal adjustments produced marked improvement. Chiropractic treatment was more effective for the wide range of symptoms common in the "neurological dysfunction syndrome," in which 13 symptom and problem areas were considered. When the problems of hyperactivity and attention span were measured statistically, chiropractic was 20 percent to 40 percent more effective than commonly used medication, with none of the adverse effects caused by drugs.

These findings are impressive, but chiropractic should not be seen as a panacea for emotional problems. Factors such as heredity, childhood conditioning, diet, and environment all play a role in mental health. Anxiety, hyperactivity, and mental illness have reached epidemic proportions in this country. The major "pseudosolution" has been the use of prescribed tranquilizers and other dangerous drugs. Because chiropractic works to restore and maintain the integrity of the nervous system, which in turn helps us to adapt better to the stresses of daily life, chiropractic can be an effective form of preventive mental-health care. In addition to being used in conjunction with therapeutic approaches—such as psychoanalysis, bioenergetics, meditation, and neurolinguistic programming (NLP)—chiropractic can offer new possibilities for aiding in the prevention and treatment of emotional problems.

Chiropractic for Special Needs

Over the years, chiropractic has provided major benefits for a number of groups with specialized needs: athletes, dancers, older adults, pregnant women, and babies and children. In the following pages we will briefly explore some of these benefits, and show how chiropractic provides a safe and natural form of both preventive and maintenance health care.

Chiropractic and the Athlete

From high school to the Olympics, chiropractic has proven to be of benefit to thousands of athletes. It is used preventively to avoid injury, to keep the athlete in top condition, or as a simple, effective form of treating such injuries as sprains, strains, and contusions. Boxers, long-distance runners, tennis players, high jumpers, cyclists, and football players have experienced the benefits of chiropractic.

Many well-known sports figures, including Tracy Austin, Roberto Clemente, and Rocky Marciano, have been counted among its devoted fans.

Active sports can place incredible strain on the body. In addition to increased stress placed on the spinal discs from running and jumping, nerve trauma can result from contusions and lacerations. Spinal nerves also can become stretched or pinched as a result of sprains, pulls, and trauma to the neck and back. Sports chiropractor Ray Horan notes: "Often, athletic injuries are caused by improper biomechanics or muscular imbalances within the spine. The spine is the essential axis of everything: The arms attach to it, the head and legs attach to it, and two-thirds of the body's muscles attach to it." According to Dr. Horan, a sport that overuses one side of the body, such as tennis, can create structural imbalances that can result in pain and muscle deficiency.

Because sports chiropractors tend to examine the entire body structure rather than confine their analysis to the obviously injured part, they can often detect an injury that would otherwise be overlooked or ignored. For example, a fall during a football game may have been heavy enough to displace a knee cartilage, but it also may have knocked the pelvis out of normal alignment. The pelvic misalignment may have more serious long-term effects than the injured knee. In addition, if the pelvis is in proper alignment, it may facilitate the healing of the knee itself.

Although chiropractors have been adjusting the spines of athletes for decades, Dr. Leroy Perry was the first to draw national attention to his work with Olympic and professional athletes. According to an article in *Sports Illustrated*, his patients have included Olympic team members such as gold-medal runner Alberto Juantorena of Cuba, high jumper Dwight Stones, skier Suzy Chaffee, football players Alex Karras and Ricky Bell, and baseball players Rick Monday, Don Sutton, and Jim Palmer. Tennis pros

Stan Smith and Tracy Austin are also counted among Dr. Perry's patients. Jimmy Connors, Billie Jean King, John McEnroe, Brad Gilbert, and Ivan Lendl are other tennis greats who have received chiropractic adjustments while in training and on tour.

Because chiropractors are experts in the field of biomechanics, they are very aware of proper posture and movement. By observing an athlete in action, a chiropractor can take note of a structural problem that can lead to injury or poor performance. For example, an incorrectly positioned seat on a racing cycle may place tension on spinal muscles and pull the vertebrae out of alignment. A tennis racquet that is too short may cause spinal nerve compression, which can produce symptoms of tennis elbow. In Dr. Perry's consultations with Stan Smith, for example, he suggested that Smith play left-handed rather than right-handed. As a result, Smith's back pain was relieved considerably.

When the cause of nerve interference and other structural problems is removed through chiropractic care, the athlete becomes stronger and better coordinated, and can better adapt to stress. As a result, he or she has a greater chance of achieving optimum performance. According to Dr. Perry, "Not only can chiropractic solve a lot of the pain and instability problems of the athlete, but the same premise that applies to rehabilitation then becomes preventive. The end result is that you enhance the performance of the athlete."

Sports chiropractic has become a specialty among many practitioners. The U.S. Olympic Committee's Advisory Council has voted unanimously to include chiropractors on all of the teams, and a growing number of sports chiropractors now work—officially and unofficially—with athletes competing in Olympic events. Many are affiliated with both amateur and professional football, hockey, basketball, soccer, baseball, track, and rugby teams. For example, Dr. Nicholas J. Athens has been the resident chiropractor for the San Francisco 49ers football team, and many give him credit for helping the team win the 1989 Super Bowl.

The American Chiropractic Association sponsors a Council of Sports Injuries and Physical Fitness, and certifies practitioners as Chiropractic Sports Physicians. In addition to traditional adjustments, most sports chiropractors employ physical therapy, which can include heat treatments, electrotherapy, ultrasound, massage, and hydrotherapy. Some offer nutritional therapy and motivational counseling as well.

Chiropractic and the Dancer

Much of what was said about chiropractic care for athletes can also be said for dancers. Like athletes, dancers are subject to a wide variety of physical, emotional, and chemical stresses due to pain-killing medications, environmental pollution, and devitalized foods. The work of a dancer involves running, jumping, placing the body in unusual or unnatural positions, and, for male dancers, heavy lifting. Repetitive movements can create muscular and structural imbalances, which can lead to vertebral subluxations. For many dancers, the rigors of competition, performance, constant practice, economic difficulties, and other pressures are sources of tremendous emotional stress. When dancers are on tour, they often have difficulty getting proper sleep and nutrition. Whether due to physical, emotional, or chemical reasons, subluxations are common among dancers. As a result, nerve compression and impingement are common afflictions. In addition to the potential for organic disease, nerve interference can affect the proper functioning of muscles, which can lead to the increased likelihood of injury and impaired peak performance.

Like sports chiropractors, those who work with dancers

are interested in how incorrect use of the body in class, rehearsals, or warm-up can contribute to poor posture and spinal misalignment. They also take into account life-style habits, such as adaptation to stress, nutrition, and rest. Some chiropractors, such as Dr. Jay Okin of New York City, recommend specific exercises both for prevention and rehabilitation. As in sports, chiropractic for dancers involves specialized knowledge and training. For this reason, it is recommended that dancers and athletes who are interested in chiropractic care seek out a practitioner who has had extensive experience in these areas.

Chiropractic and the Older Adult

Many people of retirement age have discovered that regular chiropractic care can help keep them active and healthy in their later years. Once I presented a talk to a senior citizens group. Afterward, several members of the audience told me about the dramatic benefits they experienced with a local chiropractor (whom I later consulted for my own chiropractic care). "Dr. Carl helped my arthritis." "Chiropractic helped reduce my blood pressure and my medical doctor took me off medication." "Before I found chiropractic, I had to use a cane because of my sciatica." These comments are typical of older adults who turned to chiropractic as an adjunct or alternative to conventional medical care.

Chiropractic is especially important to seniors because as a person gets older the muscles that maintain the normal alignment of the spine lose their muscle tone. As a result, the vertebrae have a greater tendency to become misaligned and hence affect the spinal nerves leading to the major organs, joints, muscles, and other tissues of the body. Serious problems such as arthritis, hypertension, constipation, and other degenerative disorders may result from an impaired nervous system.

This method of health care is gaining popularity among older adults, especially in the retirement communities in California and Florida. It is painless, both corrective and preventive, and reasonably priced. When performed with care and precision (chiropractors take account of the older adult's more fragile bones), regular chiropractic adjustments insure an uninterrupted nerve supply to keep every part of the body functioning at optimal level for the longest possible time.

Chiropractic during Pregnancy

Because additional weight and stress are placed on women during pregnancy, spinal subluxations and misalignments involving the pelvis are likely to occur. For this reason, chiropractic is often used to help lower the incidence of pain in the lower back, legs, and shoulders.

A Swedish study addressed the problem of sacroiliac pain among pregnant women. Because the increasing weight of the fetus places stress on spinal muscles, sacroiliac pain affects approximately half of all pregnant women and causes extreme discomfort. According to an article published in *Obstetrics Gynecology*, spinal manipulation helped 7 out of 10 of the women who participated in the study. Pregnant women also have reported fewer headaches, better elimination, and fewer bouts of nausea with regular chiropractic care. Very often women suffer back pain after the baby is born. A study in Italy found that postpartum pain was relieved in 90 of 120 patients who received chiropractic adjustments.

Chiropractic care during pregnancy is safe, and is sometimes administered right up to the day of birthing. However, like others with special needs, pregnant women who visit a chiropractor should be sure that he or she has experience caring for expectant mothers.

Chiropractic for the Baby or Child

Already used by older adults, chiropractic is becoming popular for young children. Since the spine is subject to frequent strain from birth through a child's accident-prone formative years, a growing number of parents are making sure their children receive chiropractic care as early as possible. Some chiropractors, such as Dr. Todd Herold, devote the bulk of their practice to the care of infants and small children.

The Birth Trauma: The First Subluxation. Perhaps the most serious cause of early subluxation is the birthing process. Unlike earlier, more natural methods that utilized midwives and birthing stools, modern hospital births (which are often easier on the doctor and harder on the baby) can involve the pulling, stretching, and twisting of the infant's body. Very often the baby's legs are forcibly extended and the rump is slapped to make the baby cry.

Emergency interventions during delivery can result in severe subluxation as well as possible brain damage. According to Arno Burnier, D.C., "The baby finds himself trapped in the birth canal. . . . For every second that the baby's cranial blood vessels are clamped down, there is anoxia [lack of oxygen] to the brain, along with various degrees of brain damage." When this occurs, the obstetricians are forced to extract the baby by means of a cesarean section or with the use of forceps.

The seriousness of spinal injuries at birth has been ignored by medical doctors until fairly recently. Abraham Towbin, M.D., affiliated with the Harvard University Medical School, reported in 1969 that spinal cord and brain stem injury is present in up to 33 percent of newborn deaths. This translates as 20,000 infant fatalities a year in this country alone. Dr. Towbin wrote:

Mechanical stress imposed by obstetrical manipulation—even the application of standard orthodox procedures—may prove intolerable to the fetus. . . . Forceful longitudinal traction during delivery, particularly when combined with flexion and torsion of the vertebral axis, is thought to be the most important cause of neonatal spinal injury.

Most children do not die at birth from such injuries, although they may well be a factor in Sudden Infant Death Syndrome (SIDS) or other life-threatening conditions during the first year of life. Strong evidence from medical literature suggests that spinal cord and brain stem injury with subluxation may cause hypoxia or chronic hypoxemia that can lead to crib death.

A case in point involved Edward Gasser of Dixon, Illinois, in September 1942. He suffered a severe asthmatic attack with respiratory failure at eight months of age. Since no medical doctor was available, his mother summoned a local chiropractor, who happened to be blind. She related the dramatic incident years later:

Around 6 in the morning Eddie turned blue, his breath stopped right below the breastbone. I had heard about this blind chiropractor, Dr. Bend, and called him. He and his assistant came right away. After feeling around his body he said: "I cannot treat a baby that small. I might kill him." . . . Ed could hardly breathe and I begged him to try, assuring him that he would surely die anyway. His assistant pleaded also, so he held Ed up toward his shoulder, holding the baby's head in his right hand, and twisted it. I heard a click and gradually Ed started breathing better. Dr. Bend's head was drenched in perspiration while he kept Eddie's head firmly in the same position for a half an hour.

He explained that the little bone in the spine that got out of place was no bigger (in a baby less than a year old) than an old-fashioned pinhead and that it was a matter of time until nature would make this bone stay put. . . . I am grateful to him as long as I live.

At the time of this writing, Edward had just celebrated his forty-eighth birthday and has not suffered an asthma attack in forty-seven years.

Although not as dramatic as the case above, thousands of newborn babies may suffer from a variety of persistent nerve defects in their early years caused by spinal injury and misalignment. Paralysis, muscle imbalance leading to poor coordination, respiratory problems, symptoms of cerebral palsy, mental retardation, epilepsy, cardiac arrhythmia, and a host of subtle nervous disorders may be present. For this reason, chiropractors suggest that babies and small children receive spinal examinations as early as possible in order to detect subluxations and other problems.

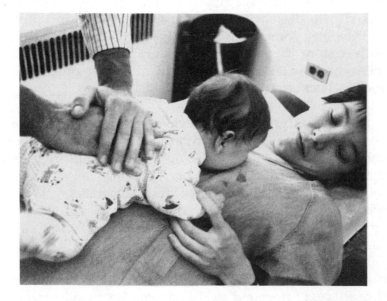

Figure 1–2. A growing number of parents want to keep their children's spines subluxation-free. Here, a baby receives a chiropractic adjustment as the parent looks on. (Courtesy of Todd Herold, D.C.)

Many infant health problems have responded well to chiropractic care. In 1985, the Danish Chiropractors Association reported that among infants suffering from infant colic, 54 percent were cured and 37 percent improved with chiropractic care. Nine percent showed no change and none were worse. Allergy, bronchial disorders, bed-wetting (among older children), asthma, Still's disease (a form of arthritis in children), and hyperactivity are other problems that have responded well to chiropractic adjustments in babies and small children.

Scoliosis. Scoliosis—a lateral *S*-shaped curvature of the spine—is estimated to affect 18 percent to 22 percent of children. Sufferers often have one shoulder higher than the other, with an accompanying pelvic tilt. Scoliosis may put pressure on nerves and internal organs, and has been linked with digestive, breathing, and childbearing problems in later years. Chiropractic is effective in helping the body restore its proper posture through regular adjustments and the possible addition of adjunctive procedures such as heel lifts.

As children grow, chiropractors advise a regular preventive program of examination and spinal care. If your children are active (and most are), they will absorb more than their share of falls, jolts, jars, sprains, and strains in the home and outdoors. Poor posture habits, sitting at school desks, and lounging in front of the television cause spinal pressure on sensitive nerves, setting the stage for serious problems later in life.

Most subluxations are corrected through the normal movement of the spine, but serious misalignments call for the services of an expert. A chiropractor is specially trained to determine if your child has any of these problems. He or she is the only practitioner qualified to correct them with safe, painless, and effective adjustments.

CHAPTER 2

Chiropractic: What It Is and What It's Not

Nearly everyone has heard of chiropractic—more than 13 million Americans used it in 1989. Yet many are unfamiliar with the theory behind it. Some believe that chiropractic is intended primarily to treat stiff necks and sore backs. Others believe that it can cure any disease known to humanity, including cancer and AIDS. Still others have trouble distinguishing chiropractic from conventional medical therapy except that medical doctors use drugs and surgery whereas chiropractors do not. Chiropractic is also confused with health systems such as osteopathy, physical therapy, acupressure, and massage.

There is no doubt that much of the confusion people have about chiropractic is due to misinformation on the part of organized medicine and its allies. However, the chiropractic profession also must accept some responsibility for the conflicting views presented to the public about its philosophy and practice. In this chapter I will attempt to clarify these issues. With the help of original material taken from the writings of D. D. Palmer, B. J. Palmer, and others, we will explore why chiropractic is a distinct and unique healing art that can revolutionize our approach to personal health care today.

Foundation of Chiropractic

In 1895, it was well known that the central nervous system—brain, spinal cord, and nerves—controls the entire body. The brain generates energy, the energy is directed down the spinal cord in the form of electrical impulses or "messages," and these *mental impulses* leave the spine at various points between the vertebrae to travel along nerve pathways to organs and tissues where they guide every function.

There is a return cycle in the nervous system as well. The brain receives a continuous stream of information from all parts of the body regarding such varied functions as digestion, repair, elimination, protection, regulation of body temperature, and the circulation of blood. With an efficiency, economy, and precision far exceeding that of the most advanced computer, the brain responds to these needs immediately and simultaneously without our being aware of it. This amazing process is essential for our survival.

Daniel David (D. D.) Palmer, the founder of chiropractic, believed that we should pay special attention to the spinal column because it contains and protects the spinal cord through which these impulses flow. He maintained that misalignments and especially subluxations of the vertebrae could impinge on the nerves branching out from the spinal cord, thus reducing their ability to supply organs or tissues with the correct amount of energy to function properly. He explained his unique premise in his book *The Science, Art and Philosophy of Chiropractic (The Chiropractor's Adjustor):*

> Displacement of any part of the skeletal frame may press against nerves, which are channels of communication, intensifying or decreasing their carrying capacity, creating either too much or not enough functioning, an aberration known as disease. The nature of the affection [effect] depends on the shape of the bone, the amount of pressure, age of patient, character of nerves impinged upon and individual makeup.

The Body Wisdom of Chiropractic: Innate Intelligence

Though Palmer's theory is now accepted by modern science, it was considered highly unorthodox in 1895. With it, he introduced a still more radical concept that continues to be a source of controversy among mainstream physicians and even some chiropractors: *innate intelligence.*

Innate intelligence is variously known in Western thought as inborn wisdom, body wisdom, the God within, organism consciousness, and living force. Millions of people sense the presence of innate intelligence, though it cannot be measured by scientific instruments. It directs the body to heal itself when sick or injured. It directs the liver to perform more than five hundred different functions in twenty-four hours without our conscious thought. It stands behind our instinct to survive and adapt to a changing environment.

Our ability to make wise judgments according to the rules of common sense also is guided by innate intelligence. D. D. Palmer explained it in the following way: "There is an inborn intelligence in every living being, and in every plant that grows. Innate [intelligence] uses the sympathetic nervous system as channels through which to transmit its orders. . . . Innate [intelligence] has all to do with the control of the vital functions, and through them, indirectly, the control of the intellectual functions."

The complement to innate intelligence is *educated intelligence.* Bartlett Joshua (B. J.) Palmer, the son of the founder and who is credited with being the developer of chiropractic, wrote: "The intelligence of the educated mind is wholly acquired—learned by experience. The innate is not acquired. It is born within us and with us, and is capable of running all functions of the body at birth as in adult life."

Chiropractors who adhere to the Palmers' philosophy

recognize the importance of educated intelligence because it is crucial to chiropractic analysis and technique. It also enables them to perform their task as practitioners, which involves a great deal of acquired knowledge and professional skill. Followers of the Palmers often express a profound respect for the body and the inborn wisdom it contains. They stress that their primary task is not to stimulate or inhibit the workings of innate intelligence like those who use drugs, heat, cold, manipulation, or surgery, but rather to *remove interference* so that the inborn wisdom can perform, unimpeded, the task of keeping the body healthy.

The Role of the Chiropractor: The Debate

D. D. Palmer defined the practitioner's unique, specialized role as the locating, analyzing, and removing of subluxations. "Chiropractors adjust, by hand, all displacements of the 200 bones, more especially those of the vertebral column, for the purposes of removing nerve impingements which are the cause of deranged functions. . . . By so doing, normal transmission of nerve-force is restored."

He believed that 95 percent of all diseases are the result of slightly displaced vertebrae and that the remaining 5 percent result from misaligned joints elsewhere in the body. B. J. Palmer at first affirmed his father's contention about skeletal misalignments, but later refined it to include only the vertebrae of the spine. He felt that limiting attention to the human spine was *the* feature that made chiropractic separate and distinct from other health-care systems. He wrote: "Chiropractors limit practice to the adjustment, by hand only, of the articulations of the human spinal column for the purpose of removing interference to the transmission of nerve energy between brain and body."

Both Palmers taught that a chiropractic adjustment is not the same as manipulation. Traditionally, a chiropractic adjustment is the application of a rapid, sudden, and precise force to a specific point of the vertebra *with the primary intention of allowing the body to remove nerve interference.* The body's reaction to the applied force realigns structure as a secondary effect. As we saw earlier, a manipulation is often a nonspecific, generalized procedure that mobilizes joints, increases their range of movement, or realigns joint structure in order to stimulate or inhibit body functions. For example, a practitioner who massages and then twists the head and neck in order to bring about a greater range of movement to the neck and skull would be performing a manipulation.

Conservative members of the chiropractic profession still utilize the traditional definition for *adjustment* to describe their work, but the distinction between manipulation and adjustment has become blurred. Among medical scientists and more liberal members of the chiropractic profession, adjustment is often referred to as *spinal manipulative therapy* or *SMT.* Although classifying the chiropractic adjustment as manipulation, the American Chiropractic Association makes the following distinction:

> Allopathic manipulation is usually little more than putting a joint through its normal range of motion, by a therapist, in order to stretch muscles or break adhesions. Osteopathic manipulation is designed to increase motion and relieve fixations. On the other hand, chiropractic corrective adjustment is made only after careful analysis, delivered in a specific manner, to achieve a predetermined goal. It is a precise, delicate maneuver, requiring special bioengineering skills.

The vast majority of chiropractic adjustments today are made on the spinal column, but some involve related structures like the pelvis. An additional technique involves light-touch reflex adjustments, which are applied to various parts of the body and are designed to reduce nerve interference. Several types of these adjustments are described in chapter 7.

D. D. Palmer's belief that all disease was a result of skeletal displacements produced much controversy in both medical and chiropractic circles. Over the years, many chiropractors either have partially disavowed his claim or have attempted to clarify his position. The noted chiropractor Hugh B. Logan, who founded the Logan College of Chiropractic and developed the famous Logan Basic Technique (described in chapter 7), offered a very sensible interpretation: "Disease is a very broad term, intended to describe not only the subjective and objective symptoms, but also all degrees of destruction or affection [sic] of tissue."

B. J. Palmer decided to discard the term *disease* from the chiropractic lexicon completely. His controversial stand centered around his belief that the primary task of the chiropractor is not the diagnosis or treatment of disease, but the elimination of subluxations: the cause of what he called *dis-ease*. *Dis-ease* is the hyphenated form of *disease*, to emphasize the original derivation meaning "lack of ease." Palmer defined *dis-ease* as "that condition which allows illness (or disease) to exist: it is dis-order or mis-alignment." Like modern holistic physicians, he pointed out that health does not imply merely the absence of disease symptoms, but a state where the body is in a state of "ease" and balance. He claimed that symptoms are often the final result of a prolonged state of dis-ease, during which an alteration of body functions has existed. For this reason, B. J. Palmer stressed the preventive aspects of chiropractic, whose goal is to focus primarily on positive wellness rather than the diagnosis and treatment of symptoms. He wrote:

> Chiropractic is a science of the cause of things natural; not a science of symptoms; not a science to chemically analyze the constituents of the human body (normal or abnormal). But it

is the science of how to analyze certain conditions quickly back to the cause, and we only utilize conditions in so far as they exist as a guidepost or mile-post on the road, telling us purely which way we must go.

B. J. Palmer was not the first to speak of chiropractic as a form of preventive health care. Just fifteen years after he discovered chiropractic, D. D. Palmer wrote, "In the near future, chiropractic will be as much valued for its preventive qualities as it is now for adjusting and relieving the cause of ailments." His belief was shared in a recent article in *Science* magazine, which said, "Allopathy is geared toward cure, while chiropractic is much more in the preventive mode."

Today, some practitioners (known as "straights") maintain the conservative philosophy set forth by the Palmers and devote their preventive efforts to manual adjustments of the vertebral column. But the majority of chiropractors (whom D. D. Palmer referred to as "mixers") hold a more liberal view. They feel that a chiropractor should be interested in all the factors that influence good health. According to the American Chiropractic Association, which represents the majority of liberal chiropractors, "Doctors of chiropractic are physicians who consider man as an integrated being, but give special attention to spinal mechanics, musculoskeletal, neurological, vascular, nutritional, and environmental relationships." In addition to spinal adjustments, their practice may include other types of manipulation of the spine, nutritional and psychological counseling, physiotherapy, first aid, and adjunctive procedures such as acupressure, soft tissue manipulation (massage), heat therapy, cold therapy, electrotherapy, and vitamin supplements to relieve pain or to assist in the body's healing process. Where permitted by law, some chiropractors can dispense nonprescription drugs and perform minor surgery. Not all liberal chiropractors utilize

these procedures, as each chiropractor sets the parameters
for his or her individual practice.

Chiropractic Defined

Because of these philosophical differences,
several definitions of chiropractic have evolved over the
years. The House of Delegates of the American Chiropractic Association (ACA) has defined chiropractic along
the original lines of D. D. Palmer to involve the entire
musculoskeletal system and not the spine alone:

> Chiropractic is that science and art which utilizes the inherent
> recuperative powers of the body and the relationship between
> the musculoskeletal structures of the body, particularly the
> spinal column and the nervous system, in the restoration and
> maintenance of health.

The conservative International Chiropractors Association (ICA) focuses more on the spinal column and immediate articulations (such as the pelvis) only:

> Chiropractic is that science and art which utilizes the inherent
> recuperative powers of the body, and deals with the rela-
> tionship between the nervous system and the spinal column,
> including its immediate articulations, and the role of this re-
> lationship in the restoration and maintenance of health.

The even more conservative Federation of Straight Chiropractic Organizations (FSCO) formally adopted the following definition of "straight chiropractic," which it believes
is more in line with the Palmers' teachings of innate intelligence and the spinal column:

> Straight chiropractic is a vitalistic philosophy of life and health
> based upon the recognition that living things have an innate

striving to maintain health, and is the art and science of correcting vertebral subluxations in accordance with that philosophy.

Of special interest is the term *vitalistic*. As opposed to mechanistic philosophy, which teaches that we are only the sum of our individual parts, vitalism teaches that there is "something else" that makes us greater than the sum of our individual parts. Vitalism is said to embrace the intangible within us that connects us to the universe. This aspect addresses the mystical approach to chiropractic that was so prevalent in early chiropractic history.

Despite these philosophical differences, there are many more points of agreement than contention within the chiropractic profession. The following points make up the essential core of chiropractic philosophy today:

1. The nervous system is of paramount importance in the body's ability to maintain itself in good health.
2. Nerve interference can diminish the body's defensive capabilities and its ability to adapt to internal or external stress and changes in the environment.
3. Spinal segments, or vertebrae, can become subluxated (misaligned).
4. Subluxation/misalignment can either directly or indirectly alter nerve messages to or from the brain, which may result in control center (brain) misinterpretation of proper function.
5. A force applied to the spine in the opposite direction of the subluxation/misalignment will allow the body's inherent recuperative powers to realign the appropriate spinal segment. The repositioning of the vertebra will result in the reduction of nerve interference, which will directly or indirectly affect the functioning of the nervous system as a whole.
6. The primary goal of a chiropractor is to adjust spinal subluxations/misalignments with the intention of re-

moving nerve interference so that optimum nerve function can be restored, thus allowing the body to effect its own cure.

This foundation has made chiropractic a unique and specialized health-care system, which has helped millions of people around the world preserve and recover their health without the use of drugs or surgery.

What Chiropractic Is Not

Many people confuse chiropractic with osteo- pathy, as well as with certain health systems often used as adjuncts to chiropractic—acupressure, massage, and physical therapy, for example. To help clarify the situation, let's review the definition and scope of each of these health systems.

Osteopathy

Chiropractic and osteopathy are often confused with each other, and with good reason: Each holds that structural derangements, especially of the spine, can lead to ill health; and both seek to realign those bones to their normal po- sition in order to restore normal body functions.

Osteopathy was founded in 1874 by Andrew Taylor Still, a surgeon from Kansas City. Still's basic premise was a simple one: the body cannot function properly unless it is structurally sound. He maintained that "all diseases are mere effects, the cause being a partial or complete failure of the nerves to properly conduct the fluids of life." He insisted that the secret to health lay in the liberation and purification of the bloodstream. As long as the blood was flowing normally, disease could not take hold. This "rule of the artery" is one feature that sets it apart from chiro- practic, which concentrates on nerve interference.

Both the osteopath and chiropractor work with misaligned bones, but they differ in their approach. Whereas chiropractic stresses manual adjustments characterized by the "dynamic thrust" applied to specific vertebrae, osteopathic manipulation is a more generalized procedure that uses leverage, traction, and pressure in order to correct abnormal structure. By structure, Still meant not only the skeleton, but the muscles, fascia (the bands or sheets of fibro-elastic tissue that envelope the whole body beneath the surface of the skin), organs, and skin. For this reason, osteopaths traditionally have employed techniques to eliminate symptoms and mobilize the body's inherent resistance to disease. These techniques include massage, stretching, twisting, and the application of water (hydrotherapy), heat, and medication.

D. D. and B. J. Palmer both were upset by the confusion of the two health systems. B. J. Palmer once reported that his father met with Dr. Still at a "bonesetter's summit" in Missouri during 1907, and the two engaged in a heated argument that attracted a large crowd. In his colorful style, the younger Palmer expressed the major differences in his textbook, *The Science of Chiropractic*:

> The osteopath, by rubbing, kneading, pressing, and a general overhauling, by neck-twisting, arm and leg wrings, aims to inhibit or stimulate nerves, whip up circulation, slow up or stimulate the action of the heart and other organs. The M.D.'s try to produce precisely the same effect by drugs. Chiropractors never deaden, inhibit or stimulate nerves, or the vital organs of the body; they free nerves from impingement, so that their impulses may be normal.

Still's claims of 100 percent cures, and his inability to explain to the satisfaction of those in conventional medicine how osteopathy worked, resulted in its banishment—like chiropractic—to professional exile, far adrift from the mainstream of medical practice.

After Still's death in 1917, refinements and modifications

of his original ideas were introduced. Osteopathy slowly began moving closer to orthodox medicine by placing more emphasis on drugs and less on manual manipulation, until it is now a semirespected (though small) part of the medical mainstream, especially in the United States. Modern osteopathic therapy can include surgery, physiotherapy, radium treatments, nutritional therapy, and drugs.

Acupressure

Acupressure (known as *Shiatsu* in Japan) is closely related to acupuncture but involves applying firm pressure of the fingertips to specific contact points (of which there are 102) rather than puncturing them with needles.

Sometimes used as an adjunct to chiropractic, acupressure is not necessarily compatible with the former's traditional approach to health. Both systems work with the inherent recuperative forces of the body, but acupressure—like acupuncture—works to stimulate the flow of energy to organs and tissues. According to the Palmers, the chiropractor's main goal is not to inhibit or stimulate, but to remove nerve interference on a fundamental level so that innate intelligence can send nerve impulses unimpeded to all the body's organs and tissues.

Applied Kinesiology

One recent development in the health field is applied kinesiology (AK), a form of preventive care developed by George Goodheart, D.C. His technique was simplified by John F. Thie, a chiropractor, who called it "Touch for Health."

Applied kinesiology does not treat specific diseases. It helps locate and correct imbalances in the body's energy system through muscles relating to the body's twelve major organs. It also can determine whether the imbalance is nutritional, psychological, or structural. To analyze a problem, the AK tester puts pressure on an arm or leg while the subject resists. If the subject cannot resist, the related organ is determined to be weak. Firm pressure is then applied to the appropriate acupuncture reflex point, stimulating the weakened area. After several moments, the muscle is retested.

Applied kinesiology has been confused with chiropractic because it is sometimes used to evaluate the effectiveness of adjustments. After the first muscle test, a chiropractic adjustment is given. A follow-up test can determine if the adjustment has helped the organ regain a normal level of function.

Physical Therapy

Physical therapy (or physiotherapy) is an established branch of medical science and is generally conducted under medical supervision. Its primary goals are to increase or restore the ability of the patient's body or body parts to perform normal activities. According to the Handbook of Physical Therapy, its objectives include increasing the range of motion of joints, correcting postural deviations, decreasing pain and swelling, and decreasing muscle spasm and spasticity. Modalities used to achieve these objectives can include moist hot packs, cold compresses, infrared heat therapy, massage, hydrotherapy, electrotherapy, corrective exercises, ultrasonic therapy, and drugs.

Unlike chiropractic, physical therapy involves the stimulation or the inhibition of body functions through the procedures employed by the practitioner. He or she decides what the patient's body needs and administers the appropriate treatment. In contrast, the primary goal of chiropractic is to remove nerve interference, so that the body's own recuperative powers can function at an optimum level.

With the exception of prescribing medications, many chiropractors (especially those who work with athletes and dancers) perform physical therapy as an adjunct to chiropractic adjustments. Qualified chiropractors often make excellent physical therapists, and many states allow them to practice physical therapy if they wish. However, it should not be confused with chiropractic itself.

Cranial Therapy

Cranial therapy was first introduced by an osteopath in the 1940s, and today it is used at times by both osteopaths and chiropractors. The goal of cranial therapy is to remove obstructions to the flow of cerebrospinal fluid, which nourishes the nerves, carries away impurities, and promotes nerve transmission throughout the body. Although it flows primarily along the spinal cord (as explained in chapter 4), it also flows along the wall of the skull. It is affected by any abnormal pressure that may occur if the bony plates of the skull are too close or too far apart.

In theory, cranial therapy works to realign the cranial bones when they are slightly out of position as a result of injury or stress. The practitioner gently palpates the area at the base of the skull—as well as the skull itself—to determine which bones are out of alignment. When the misalignments are located, the practitioner gently adjusts the bones, with the intent to restore the normal flow of the cerebrospinal fluid. This is believed to have a beneficial effect on the eyes, ears, facial muscles, and other organs and tissues serviced by nerves within the skull. Some chiropractors use cranial therapy as an adjunct to chiropractic care.

Massage Therapy

People often have a misconception that chiropractic is a form of massage. Though massage is sometimes used as an adjunct to chiropractic adjustments, the two are different.

The person skilled in massage works with soft tissues, such as muscles, fatty tissue, and skin. A massage therapist is trained in the art of kneading, slapping, rolling, pressing, and stroking these soft tissues to enable the body's self-healing process to take place. Massage can also involve increasing the mobility of joints. It is possible that massage (especially deep tissue massage) can remove nerve interference, but that is not its major goal.

Some chiropractors use massage ancillary to adjustments; others hire certified massage therapists to treat their patients before or after a chiropractic adjustment is given.

Allopathy and Chiropractic: Comparing the Basics

The principle of allopathy (conventional Western medicine) is one of the simplest known to humanity, and it makes up the foundation of the medical profession today. Unlike chiropractic, allopathy maintains that when the body's workings deviate from normal, a counteracting procedure should be applied. For example, a medical doctor would give you an alkaline for acid indigestion, a sleeping pill to treat insomnia, or a cold compress to reduce a fever. This confrontational aspect of healing is often reflected in the language of medical doctors: drugs are part of a "therapeutic arsenal," specific drugs are "magic bullets," we fight a "battle" against heart disease and a "war" on cancer.

Allopathic medicine is grounded in the mechanistic, materialistic model of life, which teaches that we human beings are each the *sum of our individual parts*. It also maintains that only what we can see and measure scientifically is of any value. According to Andrew Weil, M.D., "Belief, thought, emotion, and spiritual forces are phantoms to allopaths, sometimes mentioned in casual conversation but never accorded scientific relevance."

In contrast, chiropractic was founded on vitalistic principles. Although it also is grounded in science, it teaches that there is "something else" that cannot be measured with scientific instruments. This "something else" is innate intelligence. Whereas allopathic medicine holds that germs and harmful bacteria are the primary causes of disease, chiropractic maintains that a body that is unhealthy in the first place is vulnerable to bacteria and germs. The former prescribes a wide variety of drugs and surgery to inhibit or stimulate normal body functions, the latter does not. These important differences are reflected both in the nature and quality of the health care we receive from each system.

Doctors of Cause versus Doctors of Therapy

An enthusiastic woman told me her chiropractor had cured her arthritis. When I talked to him later, he would not take credit for healing her painful, swollen joints. I asked him why and received the simple answer, "Because we chiropractors don't cure disease." He said that professional healers never cure disease—only the body possesses the ability to heal itself. He sees his task as merely to help the body do its job by removing any interference to the natural healing process.

Most medical doctors would agree, citing that some 80 percent of disease is self-limiting. This means the body will cure the problem without any treatment at all. Although the chiropractor relieves pain and other disease symptoms in the course of his practice, he sees himself primarily as a doctor of *cause* whereas physicians are doctors of *therapy*. Traditionally, the chiropractor uses symptoms as a guidepost for a deeper problem (namely, the cause). The medical doctor devotes most of his or her attention to treating the symptoms themselves. This point was made emphatically by D. D. Palmer in 1910:

A chiropractor is not a therapeutist, as he is not interested in discovering or applying remedies. To be versed in therapeutics would require one to be skilled in the use and application of remedies. Chiropractors do not use remedies. Chiropractic principles are antipodal to [the opposite of] therapeutics. They are neither related nor pertain to therapeutics.

How do the allopathic and chiropractic approaches differ in practice? Headache, for example, is a symptom. Allopathic physicians use the therapy-oriented approach, prescribing painkilling drugs to relieve the ache. This may help us feel better, but the drug is covering the pain while the basic cause remains undetected. In this case, pain is a valuable indication telling us that something is wrong (lack of sleep, nervous tension, or a vertebral subluxation), yet this important inner voice is silenced by painkilling drugs.

Constipation is another common symptom treated by medical therapy. When it occurs, we take a laxative to force the body to eliminate waste. Most laxatives work by irritating the bowel and the body rejects them along with fecal matter. Unfortunately, the intestinal flora, normal bacteria so vitally needed for proper digestion, are often lost with the laxative and waste.

How would traditional chiropractors treat a headache or constipation? They wouldn't, specifically. Because chiropractic is primarily intended to deal with causes rather than symptoms, adjustments remove interference, enabling the body to resume the proper flow of nerve energy to the affected organ. Normal functioning then results. Since there are often factors besides nerve interference that can lead to a headache or constipation, the patient's diet, exercise habits, and stress load may be analyzed to see how they contribute to these disorders and what can be done to modify their effects.

How We "Get Sick"

Since the mid-nineteenth century, the medical profession has maintained that most illness is caused by germs, harmful bacteria, and viruses transmitted to people through food, breath, and touch. Our language reflects this idea, as in "catching" a cold, "coming down with a bug," or "it's been going around."

Chiropractors do not ignore the fact that environmental factors (which include germs and microbes) can be involved in the disease process. They acknowledge that germs, viruses, and bacteria play a vital role in the scheme of life. As nature's scavengers, such microorganisms thrive on weak, sick, devitalized, and dead tissue cells. To the degree that our general state of health is not reaching its potential, the weaker our resistance and the more likely we can become infected by germs and virulent strains of bacteria. This view about germs is not a chiropractic invention. On his deathbed, Louis Pasteur, the French biochemist and bacteriologist who developed the germ theory, said: "Le germe n'est rien, c'est le terrain qui est tout (The microbe is nothing, the soil is everything)." By "the soil" he meant the body, as it is the body that harbors the germs and then becomes sick.

In the healing profession, many physicians, nurses, and others find themselves in close contact with sick patients who often breathe and even cough in their faces. Nurses and orderlies have been known to work with tubercular patients for thirty years or more without ever coming down with tuberculosis. Healers such as Florence Nightingale, Albert Schweitzer, and Mother Teresa spent many years treating people suffering from the most dangerous diseases known to humanity, and yet they are remembered for their long, healthy, and productive lives. Obviously, their bodies' natural defense systems kept them healthy, rather than the control of germs and bacteria.

The immune system has the natural ability to protect us from germs and bacteria by producing antibodies and other cell defense mechanisms. Over the past decade, it has been established that the proper functioning of the immune system is determined in part by a healthy and unimpeded nervous system. For this reason, chiropractors see their primary task as working to assure the uninterrupted function of the nervous system.

No responsible chiropractor would guarantee that chiropractic care can make us immune to all germs and disease. However, instead of blaming illness on germs or "bad luck," chiropractic can play a unique role in the health-care field by insuring a strong nerve supply to every part of the body. This energy flow helps maintain all tissue cells in good health. A germ or virus does not have fertile ground on which to sustain itself when it enters a healthy, properly functioning human body.

Surgery

One of the most common functions of allopathic medicine is to recommend and perform surgery—the repair or removal of body parts or tissues by cutting. Although chiropractors never perform surgery (except in Oregon, where a chiropractor is permitted to remove warts), they believe that some operations may at times be necessary. An emergency procedure to save a life—as in the case of a seriously diseased organ, a compound fracture, a hernia repair, or bullet wound or other injury—may require an operation.

However, there is much public concern that many operations are unnecessary. According to former Health, Education, and Welfare Secretary Joseph A. Califano, Jr., there is growing consensus that half the coronary bypasses, most cesarean sections, and a significant proportion of operations such as pacemaker implants and hysterectomies are not needed.

Although chiropractors recognize the occasional need for surgery, many believe that it is difficult to enjoy total health after the surgical removal of an organ. The organs of the body function interdependently, and when one organ is surgically removed the remaining organs may not be able to fully compensate for the loss. Although people have been known to live full and active lives after surgery, their health is usually not as good as it was before they became ill. For this reason, most chiropractors stress the preventive side of their practice, which can help your body avoid a condition that may require surgery later on.

A Pill for Every Ill

The Statistical Abstract of the United States notes that Americans spent more than $30 billion in 1986 on more than 4000 different prescription and nonprescription drugs—a 350 percent increase from 1970. This includes over 6 billion doses of antibiotics a year. According to New Scientist, the annual pretax profits of the "industry leaders" among drug manufacturers can reach 40 percent.

Chiropractors do not prescribe drugs, but they believe that certain medications may be necessary to save a life or maintain certain body functions when all else fails. However, the chiropractic profession traditionally has been opposed to those medical doctors and drug companies who proclaim that they have "a pill for every ill and a potion for every emotion," and that it is perfectly all right to take a drug for every little thing that comes along.

In the United States and other industrialized nations, central nervous system drugs (barbiturates, tranquilizers, and amphetamines) represent the fastest growing sector of the pharmaceutical industry, amounting to one-third of total sales. Chiropractors are concerned about the possible effects that stimulants and tranquilizers have on the nervous system and its ability to maintain the body in optimum health and mental condition. In addition to physical and emotional effects, chemicals (such as drugs) often produce subluxations.

Chiropractors also worry about the negative side effects that drugs may have on the body in general, an example of iatrogenic disease. According to the medical textbook *Hazards of Medication*, more than 1.5 million of all people admitted to hospitals every year suffer from the side effects of drugs and medical therapy. Although drug companies rarely tell us directly, their advertisements in medical journals carry long lists of adverse reactions that can be caused by their products. Even common aspirin, which is considered among the most harmless of drugs, claims the lives of more than 1600 people a year as a result of internal hemorrhages alone, and thousands more die from other adverse reactions. According to the *Journal of the American Medical Association*, the ingestion of aspirin in doses of 1 to 3 grams a day (the most popular brand contains 6.5 grams per tablet) will induce gastrointestinal bleeding in about 70 percent of normal individuals.

Another major concern involves dangerous *synergistic* effects, which occur when two or more drugs combine in the body to produce a chemical reaction. An example of this made headlines after the sudden death of Elvis Presley in 1977. According to the medical examiner's report, ten prescription drugs were present in the singer's bloodstream when he died. The synergistic reaction they produced contributed to his death.

For the majority of individuals, drugs are taken habitually in order to relieve unpleasant symptoms. Chiropractic teaches that drugs only suppress or alter symptoms and body functions. A fever is one way the body fights off infection—if an aspirin is taken to reduce it, the body's ability to combat the infection is reduced.

Chiropractors believe that lack of sleep, emotional stress, improper diet, poor sanitation, smoking, lack of exercise, overeating, and alcohol abuse can cause subluxations and nerve interference. These factors can also contribute to pain and other symptoms. For this reason, a chiropractor's primary task is to work with nature to help normalize proper body function. Drugs cover up symptoms, cause physical and psychological dependency, and create adverse side effects. Chiropractic teaches that a move away from drugs toward the natural ability of the body to heal itself will have a positive, lasting effect on our health, which will be passed to future generations.

One final point: it is important to know that chiropractors do not totally reject conventional medicine. Often by the time symptoms appear, the "crisis care" of an allopathic physician may be more appropriate than chiropractic alone. Although chiropractors advocate the conservative health care they provide to help the body heal itself, they are trained to recognize a health problem that should receive the attention of a physician. Most refer patients to medical doctors, and many, including B. J. Palmer, have sought medical care themselves.

CHAPTER 3

Chiropractic's Controversial History

Chiropractic will celebrate its hundredth birthday in 1995, yet its roots extend back to the beginnings of recorded history. One historian cites an ancient Kong Fou document from China, written about 2700 B.C., that describes tissue manipulation. An early Greek papyrus dating back to 1500 B.C. gives instructions on maneuvering the lower extremities to treat low back conditions. Manipulation of sprained, dislocated, displaced, and crushed vertebrae was used in early Egypt. A rare surviving work, now called the *Edwin Smith Surgical Papyrus*, was studied by physicians some seventeen hundred years before Christ. The following advice helped them to make a proper diagnosis:

> If thou examinest [a man having] a sprain in a vertebra of his spinal column, thou shouldst say to him: "Extend now thy two legs [and] contract them both [again]." When he extends them both he contracts them both immediately because of the pain he causes in the vertebra of his spinal column in which he suffers.

Most of us would laugh at this test for something as obvious as back sprain, but early Egyptians may actually have discovered the complex relationship between the vertebrae, the spinal nerves, and the leg muscles.

Spinal manipulation was not limited to the Old World. It was practiced in one form or another by the Sioux, Winnebago, and Creek peoples in North America. The Incas of South America used it for illness and back pain, as did the Aztec, Toltec, Tarascan, Zoltec, and Mayan cultures of Mexico and Central America. In the Pacific region, "foot walking" was a popular form of treatment for disease and other ailments in early Polynesia, and children used to walk along the backs of their ailing elders. Even today, ancient backwalking techniques are practiced by the Maori peoples of New Zealand.

The greatest breakthrough took place in ancient Greece. The Father of Medicine, Hippocrates (460–377 B.C.), was the first physician to link spinal misalignments with ill health. His students were advised to "get knowledge of the spine, for this is the requisite for many diseases." They were taught the value and practice of special techniques described in several now-famous medical texts. In teaching a practitioner how to reduce a posterior spinal curvature caused by a fall, he wrote:

> The physician, or some person who is strong and not unin-structed, should apply the palm of one hand to the hump, and then, having laid the other hand upon the former, he should make pressure, attending whether this force should be applied directly downward, or toward the head, or toward the hips.

Hippocrates also designed the first table for making spinal adjustments, as seen in Figure 3–1. Fitted with various pulleys and clamps, his invention enabled the physician to make effective adjustments with a minimum of risk to the patient.

Many early physicians echoed Hippocrates' advice, but Claudius Galen (A.D. 129–199) stands out among them. A Greek physician who dominated medicine during the early Roman Empire, Galen was among the first to recognize the importance of the nervous system. As a result of his animal dissections (the dissection of humans was consid-

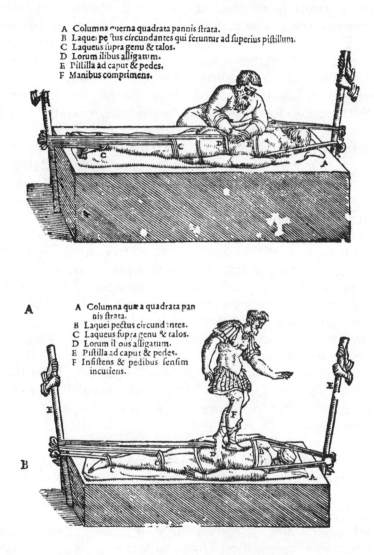

A Columna cuerna quadrata pannis ſtrata.
B Laquei pẹ ʔtus circundantes qui feruntur ad ſuperius piſtillum.
C Laqueus ſupra genu & talos.
D Lorum ilibus alligatum.
E Piſtilla ad caput & pedes.
F Manibus comprimens.

A

A Columna quæ a quadrata pan
  nis ſtrata.
B Laquei pectus circundantes.
C Laqueus ſupra genu & talos.
D Lorum il ous alligatum.
E Piſtilla ad caput & pedes.
F Inſiſtens & pedibus ſenſim
  incutiens.

B

*Figure 3–1. Top: A method of traction and sustained pressure rec-
ommended in the works of Hippocrates. Bottom: A man standing on
the sufferer's back to apply pressure in the course of traction. (Galen,
after Hippocrates; courtesy, the Wellcome Trustees)*

ered sinful), he discovered seven of the twelve important cranial nerves. The cervical, lumbar, and dorsal (*thoracic*) regions of the spine were also named and defined. Although understanding human anatomy took centuries, Galen's work had positive impact on our understanding of human health and disease. His admonition to "look to the nervous system as the key to maximum health" would have a direct impact on the development of chiropractic some seventeen hundred years later.

The fall of the Roman Empire in A.D. 476 plunged twenty centuries of accumulated human knowledge into darkness. Hundreds of libraries were plundered and thousands of scientific documents were burned by invaders. The evolution of medicine was severely curtailed during this period appropriately known as the Dark Ages. Scientific inquiry and understanding were replaced with fear and superstition. The development of spinal manipulation also was set back during this time. The popping sound so commonly heard during treatment was thought to come from demons (then accepted as the cause of disease) that were being driven from the patient. Despite this belief, the art of spinal manipulation was not lost completely. It was kept alive (often in secret) by mainly unschooled physicians throughout Europe, especially in the area known today as Germany.

By the late Middle Ages, spinal manipulation became known to the public again, and it enjoyed wide popularity throughout the Renaissance, when it was known as *bonesetting*. Using knowledge handed down from parent to child, early bonesetters were regarded as gifted healers who could treat a wide variety of illnesses, aches, and pains by manipulating bones back into place. Often successful when other treatment failed, bonesetting quickly spread throughout Europe and by the eighteenth century was one of the most recognized healing arts on the Continent.

Bonesetting didn't become popular in the United States until the following century, when it expanded with western migration. One of the most famous practitioners in this country was Steven Sweet of Sag Harbor, Long Island, the head of a famous family of bonesetters. Though he was totally untrained and lacked a basic education, he treated many ailments that were beyond the ability of even highly trained medical doctors at the time.

Interest in this skill was not limited to the "uneducated." The renowned British surgeon Sir James Paget wrote an article entitled "Cases that Bonesetters Cure" for the January 5, 1865, issue of the *British Medical Journal*. Dr. Wharton Hood of London shared his observations in his treatise *On Bonesetting*, which received wide acclaim in medical circles. "I was astounded," he wrote, "and often no less mortified, at the number and variety of instances in which the manipulations I have endeavoured to describe were followed by almost immediate cure." This success led to greater interest in the spine among medical doctors, and several scholarly works were written during the nineteenth century as a result.

The First Adjustment

It was September 18, 1895, in the middle of a busy workweek in Davenport, Iowa. Harvey Lillard, a janitor at the Putnam Building, was relating to Daniel David Palmer how he had become virtually deaf. Palmer was a magnetic healer (one that heals by laying on of hands) who practiced there. He later described this event in his book *The Science, Art and Philosophy of Chiropractic*:

> Harvey Lillard, a janitor in the Ryan Block, where I had my office, had been so deaf for 17 years that he could not hear the racket of a wagon on the street or the ticking of a watch.

I made inquiry as to the cause of his deafness and was informed that when he was exerting himself in a cramped, stooped position, he felt something give way in his back and immediately became deaf. An examination showed a vertebra racked from its normal position. I reasoned that if that vertebra was replaced, the man's hearing should be restored. With this object in view, a half-hour's talk persuaded Mr. Lillard to allow me to replace it. I racked it into position by using the spinous process as a lever and soon the man could hear as before.

After three adjustments in as many days, Lillard jumped up and cried, "Doc! Doc! I hear!" For the first time in seventeen years, Harvey Lillard could make out the rumble of the horse-drawn trolleys four stories below. This was the birth of the science of chiropractic.

D. D. Palmer: The Founder

Daniel David Palmer was born on March 7, 1845, near the town of Port Perry, Ontario, Canada. As a boy, he would often take to the woods in search of skeletons of animals that had died the winter before. Sometimes along with them he brought home a small animal with a broken bone. He would apply tiny splints fashioned of twigs and strips of cloth, and the bones often mended. His mother would say that young Daniel had "healing hands." When a member of the family was ill, they would look to him for comfort. His interest in health continued into adolescence, when Daniel spent much of his free time reading books on anatomy and how the body worked.

Palmer left Ontario in 1865 and moved to the United States with his brother, Tom. He first settled in New Boston, Illinois, where he married and became a prosperous beekeeper. After his wife's death Palmer remarried and moved to What Cheer, Iowa, where he worked as a fish peddler and grocer. Following the death of his second wife, Palmer and his three children eventually settled in the small town of Letts, Iowa, a few miles from the Mississippi River.

At this time, Palmer resumed his reading and gradually became open to new ideas in health and metaphysics. He began to teach classes in business and to lecture from town to town on the subject of phrenology, an ancient system of character analysis based on the study of the features of the skull. During a tour he met Paul Caster, an internationally known magnetic healer from nearby Burlington, Iowa. Visiting him several days later, Palmer was astounded by the collection of abandoned crutches, canes, and braces hanging on the office walls and he soon became a student of Caster's. Eventually he began his own practice in Burlington after rediscovering his early talents and interest in healing the sick.

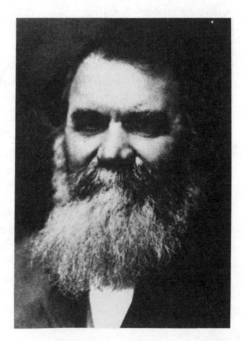

Figure 3–2. D. D. Palmer
(1845–1913)

Throughout nine years as a magnetic healer, Palmer read many books on anatomy and physiology, devoting much time to the human spine. He learned that the body receives nerve energy through the vertebral column, and that an impingement of the spinal nerves could inhibit the energy flowing from the brain through the nerves to various organs of the body. He concluded that misaligned vertebrae could well be a cause of disease.

With increasing success as a healer, Palmer shortened his name to "D. D." and began calling himself "Doctor," a rather common practice in those days. Palmer has often been ridiculed for his lack of medical training and for the fact that he worked as a grocer. However, his knowledge of anatomy surpassed that of most doctors, many of whom once worked as laborers, farmers, and businessmen themselves. Medical schools in those days required less than a year of attendance, and many of their graduates became itinerant practitioners who sold snake oil and other remedies of dubious value.

After D. D. Palmer made the dramatic discovery of chiropractic in 1895, he began to refine the technique and develop the philosophy for a new healing art. His belief that illness is essentially functional and becomes organic only as an end product is finding acceptance today in medical circles. In addition, his comments about the metaphysical aspects of health are much in tune with modern views on holistic health. He wrote:

> The human body represents the actions of three laws, spiritual, mechanical and chemical, united as one. . . . As long as there is perfect union of these three there is health. This machine, like all others, is run by power, called mental impulses, made in the brain and connected with the body by a system of nerves thru [sic] which this force passes in currents, including the higher exemplification of intellectual power. Functions are names given to these actions, any interference to the passage of these vitalizing currents produces abnormal functions—disease.

One of Palmer's most devoted patients was Rev. Samuel H. Weed, who had been successfully treated for sciatica. The minister coined the term *chiropractic* from the Greek words χειρ, "hand," and πρακτικός, "practice." In Palmer's words, a *chiropractor* is "a hand practitioner—one who repairs or one who adjusts."

A strong-willed and suspicious individual who wanted to keep chiropractic for himself and his family, Palmer was not eager to share his discovery with others. After months of persuasion by his equally strong-minded son, Bartlett Joshua (B. J.), D. D. Palmer reluctantly established the Palmer Infirmary and Chiropractic Institute in Davenport in 1897. Featuring a three-month course, the new institution attracted a diversity of students including several women, medical doctors, osteopaths, and surgeons. Among them was Dr. Alfred F. Walton of the Medical College of the University of Pennsylvania, who had graduated from Harvard University Medical School. After becoming a chiropractor, he lectured and wrote extensively in support of the new healing art, helping make it respectable in the eyes of many physicians.

B. J. Palmer: The Developer

Bartlett Joshua Palmer is hailed as the second most important figure in the history of chiropractic. Fourteen years old when the new science was founded, he helped elevate it to the second largest health-care system in America by the time he died in 1961. During his lifetime he was a brilliant and colorful chiropractor, writer, teacher, lecturer, and radio pioneer. He was also responsible for saving chiropractic from extinction in its early years and preserved many of the original principles laid down by his father. B. J. was one of the first students to graduate from his father's new school, a member of the class of 1902. B. J. often clashed with his father, and after graduation left Davenport to practice in Lake City, Iowa, West Virginia, and Michigan. While practicing in Manistique, Michigan, he received a telegram from his father to return to Davenport.

Haunted by the fear that his beloved chiropractic would become sullied by the use of adjunct therapies, D. D. Palmer grew secretive and intolerant toward other points of view. His practice had diminished and his school ceased to attract new students. By the time B. J. Palmer returned from Michigan, his father was $8000 in debt and threatened with the probable demise of his fledgling school. B. J., then only 21 years old, took over his father's affairs and D. D. left town.

After a few months the younger Palmer was well on the way to settling the debts, and the Palmer Infirmary and Chiropractic Institute began attracting students once more. At the same time, B. J. began to develop his father's ideas into a well-organized science that would build a stronger foundation for the future.

D. D. Palmer's absence from Davenport was short. When he returned, he discovered, to his surprise and resentment, that B. J. had the situation well in hand, and he reluctantly shared the administration of the school with his son. The next years were difficult for both men. The love-hate relationship between these two strong-willed personalities proved to have a major impact on the development of chiropractic and the growth of chiropractic colleges.

In 1903, the Palmers had their first taste of organized medicine's opposition to chiropractic: they were arrested for practicing medicine without a license. Although B. J. was never brought to trial, D. D. Palmer was fined $500 and remanded to prison until his son paid the fine seventeen days later. It is still unclear why B. J. was never brought to trial, but the fact that he wasn't made his father more resentful than ever.

Within a year of this incident, the Palmers decided to dissolve their partnership. The founder sold his share of the infirmary and school to his son and left Davenport to set up chiropractic schools in Oregon and Oklahoma. He also began writing his 1008-page text *The Science, Art and Philosophy of Chiropractic*, which was published in 1910. D. D. Palmer finally settled in Los Angeles, where he died in 1913, several months after being hit by a car while marching in a school parade in Davenport. The driver of the car was B. J. Palmer. Although it was never proven that B. J. was guilty of patricide, rumors persisted for many years.

In 1904, B. J. renamed the school the Palmer School of Chiropractic and moved it to what is today part of the present Palmer College campus. The school was later to be known as the "chiropractic fountain head" and would graduate the majority of the world's chiropractors. By the end of 1906, B. J. Palmer had published the first major textbook on chiropractic, *The Science of Chiropractic: Its Principles and Adjustments* (coauthored with his father, but he later claimed sole authorship in subsequent editions). He had also married Mable Heath, an early student at the P.S.C., who had studied anatomy at the Rush Medical College in Chicago. Known as the First Lady of Chiropractic, she served on the faculty of the Palmer School and played a leading role in attracting women to the profession until her death in 1949.

B. J. was embroiled in controversy for much of his life. As a man of determination who was strict in his philosophy, he incurred the wrath of many chiropractors who did not want to limit chiropractic to manual spinal adjustments. In 1906, P.S.C. faculty member John Howard left the school during a dispute over his desire to use cadavers from the local morgue for dissection. He started the National School of Chiropractic, which was later moved to Chicago.

In 1910, Palmer alienated a group of his own students and faculty by introducing the *spinograph*, the first X-ray machine ever used to detect spinal misalignments. They objected to the use of anything but hands in chiropractic analysis (Palmer believed that chiropractic *adjustments* should be limited to hands only, but chiropractic *analysis* need not). Leaving the Palmer School during one of B. J.'s classes, the group established the Universal Chiropractic College several blocks down the street. Ironically, the U.C.C. began using the spinograph and, after the college moved to Pittsburgh in 1918, its researchers invented the first X-ray machine that photographed the entire spine while the patient stood upright. As a result, spinographs could show, for the first time, the effects of unequal leg length, pelvic distortion, and body stress under the normal influence of gravity.

Fifteen years later, Palmer's introduction of the *neurocalometer* sparked another exodus of faculty and students. It was a handheld device featuring two heat-sensitive prongs designed to measure temperature differences on either side of the spine without causing pain to the patient. Because such differences can indicate the existence of nerve interference, the neurocalometer and its successors are widely used today to locate subluxations throughout the vertebral column. He also introduced his "hole-in-one" adjusting technique, which involved only the first and second cervical (*atlas* and *axis*) vertebrae. In addition to his claim that no chiropractor could practice without a neurocalometer, he said that any chiropractor who did not use his HIO technique was practicing dishonestly.

Under the influence of B. J. Palmer, chiropractic experienced rapid growth. By 1920, half of the forty-eight states had recognized chiropractic and the Canadian province of Ontario soon followed suit. Dozens of chiropractic colleges sprang up around the country. Two national organizations were established to represent the growing profession: the

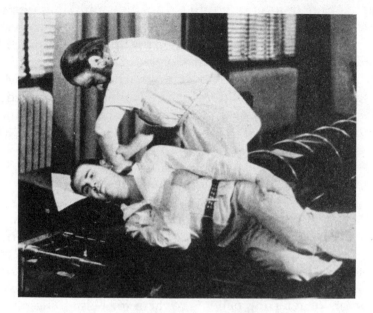

Figure 3–3. B. J. Palmer (1888–1961) performing his famous "hole-in-one" chiropractic adjustment. (Photo courtesy of the Canadian Memorial Chiropractic College)

National (now American) Chiropractic Association and the Universal (now International) Chiropractors Association, the latter founded by B. J. Palmer himself.

In addition to B. J. Palmer, other outstanding chiropractors played important roles. Dr. John J. Nugent urged chiropractors to raise their educational standards, and his efforts helped bring the profession closer to serious consideration by established academic accrediting agencies. Dr. Willard Carver, who once presided over four chiropractic schools at the same time, extended D. D. Palmer's original concepts to include the idea that nerve interference can occur in other parts of the body in addition to the spine. Carver introduced soft tissue manipulation, "mental science" (a form of positive thinking), and kinesiology into chiropractic, and he stressed the importance of correct posture. Dr. Leo J. Spears founded the Spears Chiropractic Hospital and Sanitarium in Colorado, now the world's largest hospital for intensive chiropractic care. Dr. L. M. Rogers, one-time president of the National Chiropractic Association, encouraged chiropractors to be more scientific in their approach.

Organized Medicine: The Enemy

Expansion of this new approach into primary health care alarmed the organized medical profession. The American Medical Association's first tactic was to try to isolate chiropractic. In 1933, the Judicial Council of the AMA discouraged members from consulting with chiropractors or referring patients to them for help: "The physician who maintains professional relations with cult practitioners would seem to exhibit a lack of faith in the correctness and efficacy of scientific medicine and to admit that there is merit to cult practitioners."

Another tactic was to require chiropractic students to take the Basic Science Exam that was designed for medical doctors and osteopaths. B. J. Palmer loudly condemned this rule and claimed that since chiropractic was neither medicine nor a form of medical therapy, students should not have to take an examination designed by and for the medical profession. Between 1927 and 1944 only 28 percent of chiropractic students passed and many chiropractic schools were forced to close their doors.

Palmer and his colleagues fought back to rally grassroots support for their profession. They began offering free adjustments to actors, singers, and acrobats, many of whom were helped by chiropractic and didn't hesitate to recommend it. In order to promote his ideas, Palmer started two of the earliest radio stations in the country (the call letters of WOC in Davenport supposedly stood for "Wonders of Chiropractic," and WHO in Des Moines symbolized "With Hands Only"). These and other grass-roots efforts to save chiropractic worked. By the early 1950s, the profession had resumed its steady growth, and by the early 1960s millions of Americans chose chiropractic care every year for themselves and their families.

After B. J. Palmer's death in 1961, organized medicine was more determined than ever to send chiropractic to destruction. The earlier 1933 AMA statement was changed to a firm command. Any medical doctor who associated with a chiropractor was branded as "unethical." In 1963, the AMA Board of Trustees established a Committee on Quackery to contain and eliminate the chiropractic profession. A confidential memorandum to the AMA Department of Investigation dated September 21, 1967, revealed the committee's short-range goals:

1. Doing everything within our power to see that chiropractic coverage under Title 18 of the Medicare Law is not obtained.
2. Doing everything within our power to see that recognition of listing by the U.S. Office of Education of chiropractic accrediting agency is not achieved.
3. To encourage continued separation of the two national chiropractic organizations.
4. To encourage state medical societies to take the initiative in their state legislatures in regard to legislation that might affect the practice of chiropractic.

The long-range goal was ominous: "Chiropractic licensure should be made so difficult that eventually more chiropractors are dying than new chiropractic licenses are granted." Radiologists were told that providing X-ray services to chiropractors and their patients was unethical. The Radiological Society of New York warned: "A practicing radiologist in the State of New York shall have no voluntary association with cultists of chiropractic, including consultation or the acceptance of referrals." High schools were not exempt from the conspiracy. A letter from the president of the Pennsylvania Medical Society to guidance counselors condemned chiropractic as an "unscientific cult," adding, "To direct a highly motivated and intelligent student into a career in chiropractic would indeed be a loss to society."

Chiropractic Fights Back—and Wins

Despite efforts to assure itself a health-care monopoly in the United States and to deny freedom of choice to American consumers, the AMA was unable to eliminate or even contain chiropractic. In 1974, four historic events took place that were major victories:

1. Louisiana became the last of fifty states to grant a separate board of licensure.
2. The Office of Education of the Department of Health, Education, and Welfare authorized the Council of Chiropractic Education (CCE) to begin accrediting training colleges.
3. Congress included chiropractic care in its Medicare program.
4. Congress authorized a $2 million study on the scientific basic of chiropractic, which resulted in the landmark 1975 report *The Research Status of Spinal Manipulative Therapy*. This gave practitioners equal status with other health-care professionals.

The Wilk Antitrust Suit

Two years later, an even more important event took place which would have a major impact on the future of chiropractic. In 1976, Dr. Chester A. Wilk and three other chiropractors initiated an antitrust suit against the American Medical Association, four AMA officials, and ten other medical groups, including the American College of Surgeons and the American College of Radiology. They claimed that these organizations violated the Sherman Antitrust Act by conspiring to make it difficult for them as doctors of chiropractic to exercise their right to practice and offer their services to the public.

After eleven years of intense litigation, Federal District Judge Susan Getzendanner ruled that the AMA and two other medical groups had indeed violated U.S. antitrust laws by encouraging a boycott of chiropractors in an effort to eliminate their profession. On August 28, 1987, the judge permanently barred the AMA from hindering the chiropractic profession and cited the anti-competitive effects of the defendants' actions.

[The boycott is] anti-competitive and it raises costs to interfere with the consumer's free choice to take the product of his liking; it is anti-competitive to prevent medical physicians from referring patients to a chiropractor; it is anti-competitive to impose higher costs on chiropractors by forcing them to pay for their own X-ray equipment rather than obtaining X-rays from hospital radiology departments or radiologists in private practice; and it is anti-competitive to prevent chiropractors from improving their education in a professional setting by preventing medical physicians from teaching or lecturing to chiropractors.

In addition to "labeling all chiropractors unscientific cultists and depriving chiropractors of association with medical physicians, injury to reputation was assured by the

AMA's name-calling practice." Judge Getzendanner described the conspiracy as "systematic, long-term wrongdoing and the long-term intent to destroy a licensed profession." At the time of this writing, an injunction has been issued and monetary compensation is being considered.

Today, nearly every community in the nation is served by at least one doctor of chiropractic. Enrollment in training colleges is at an all-time high, and approximately twenty-five hundred chiropractors graduate each year. An estimated 13 million people consulted the nation's thirty-five thousand chiropractors in 1989, and received approximately 163 million chiropractic adjustments. More than six hundred insurance companies provide for chiropractic care in health and accident policies. Claims are honored under Medicare, Medicaid, federal vocational rehabilitation programs, and worker's compensation programs in the United States and Canada. Sixteen out of twenty-two employee organization plans under Federal Employee Health Benefits cover chiropractic services. Millions of union members and many national employee organizations are eligible for care. Many health systems agencies (HSAs) include chiropractors as members of their boards of governors, as technical advisors, and as area council members.

Chiropractic has not only survived but flourished for almost a century because millions of people around the world have insisted on the unique service it provides. Whether used as a preventive means to insure good health, or as a way to help the body cure itself of disease, chiropractic has succeeded where other health-care measures have failed.

Is the battle over? Not quite. Despite the successful conclusion of the lawsuit, it is probable that the medical profession will continue its opposition to chiropractic. Many chiropractors fear that the next phase of the struggle will be chiropractic's gradual absorption into medical practice (as happened with the osteopathic profession), rather than its remaining a separate and distinct form of health care. Others believe that chiropractic may become a form of limited medical therapy, such as dentistry or podiatry.

There is some justification for these concerns. Over the past few years, the unique focus of chiropractic care to remove nerve interference, chiropractic's stress on health maintenance and preventive care as opposed to therapy and disease care, and the use of alternative terminology that chiropractors have traditionally preferred (such as *analysis* instead of *diagnosis*, and *adjustment* instead of *treatment*) have not received the emphasis they had in the past. In addition, a growing number of chiropractors are practicing medical modalities (such as physical therapy), which tends to blur the distinctions between the two professions. These trends will be watched closely by chiropractors and patients alike, for they will determine the type of health care we and our children will receive in the years to come.

PART TWO

Chiropractic and the Consumer

CHAPTER 4

How Chiropractic Works: The Education of the Patient

Daniel David Palmer was ridiculed by members of the medical profession when he said the normally functioning brain, operating through a sound nervous system, regulates and integrates every body activity down to the workings of the tiniest cell. Today, his theory—on which chiropractic is based—is universally accepted by the scientific community and is taught in every medical school in the country.

Every organ of the body receives its vital nerve supply from the brain via the spinal cord and nerve trunks. If the supply is interfered with, an increase or decrease of nerve energy to an organ or tissue can result. Because the central nervous system is housed by the spinal column, and communicates with every part of the body from it, the science of chiropractic has concerned itself specifically with spinal structure. It investigates how misalignments alter functions of the central nervous system and lead to ill health. Understanding how to correct nerve interference and restore proper energy transmission to the entire body is the chief goal of chiropractic. For this reason, a lay person's knowledge of the nervous system can help you become a partner with your chiropractor in maintaining your health.

Your nervous system is constantly at work. It receives, processes, and transmits messages to and from the brain and eyes, ears, nose, and skin to help the body respond to its outer environment. If you accidentally touch a hot skillet, your nervous system will tell you—in a fraction of a second and in no uncertain terms—that the extreme heat is dangerous, and that you should remove your hand.

In addition, the nervous system maintains the body's inner environment and regulates the digestion of food and the amount of carbon dioxide in the blood without your being aware of it. Whether you are moving your eyes across a page in order to read these words or secreting intestinal fluids to digest the salad you enjoyed for lunch, the nervous system is performing its tasks with lightning speed and exacting precision.

The nervous system has two main divisions. The *central nervous system (CNS)* is composed of the brain, spinal cord, and nerves as they exit from the spine. It is largely responsible for helping the body adapt to its external environment, as in locomotion and the ability to sense our surroundings. The *autonomic nervous system* is responsible for carrying out the involuntary processes of the body such as digestion, repair, and elimination. Without our conscious thought it adjusts the functions of the muscles and the internal organs to the advantage of the body as a whole.

Within the autonomic nervous system, two sets of nerves generally work opposite each other to regulate homeostasis, or body balance. One set (known as the *sympathetic nervous system*) speeds up the heart and slows down digestion; the other set (the *parasympathetic nervous system*) slows down the heart and speeds up digestion. Both systems reach nearly every tissue of the body. Together, with utmost precision, the sympathetic and parasympathetic nerves regulate the body's functions and keep them in perfect balance. They are especially important in regulating the thymus gland and the spleen, which have been found to play an important role in the immune system. These two organs manufacture lymphocytes, the white blood cells that protect us from viruses, harmful bacteria, and incipient cancers.

Both the central and autonomic nervous systems are interconnected by way of the spinal nerves. Any predisposing condition or obstruction in one system can alter the normal function of the other. A simplified drawing (Figure 4–1) reveals the major divisions and their relationships to important body organs.

Brain, Spine, and Nerves: A Team Effort

The central nervous system is of special importance to the practitioner who works to keep it free of interference. The CNS begins in the brain, which contains billions of *neurons*, or nerve cells, that transmit information from one part of the nervous system to another. If an analogy were made between the number of nerve connections in our brain and all the connecting lines of a modern telephone system, the brain would achieve more "thought combinations" than a vast network carrying all the conversations on every telephone in the world.

From the base of the brain, the spinal cord extends through the spinal column (Figure 4–2). The spinal cord is composed of millions of nerves, which the brain uses as a pathway to control and govern the function of every organ and tissue of the body. Just as the brain is protected by a reinforced shield of bone (the skull), nature has given the spinal cord special protection as well. Its first line of defense is the spinal column composed of a long series of bones called *vertebrae*. These encase the spinal cord and protect it from injury. The cord is then wrapped with a tough covering, and *cerebrospinal fluid* flows within this covering. Although we don't know everything about this unique fluid, we do know it is vital to the transmission of nerve impulses and to the proper nourishment and cleansing of delicate nerve tissue.

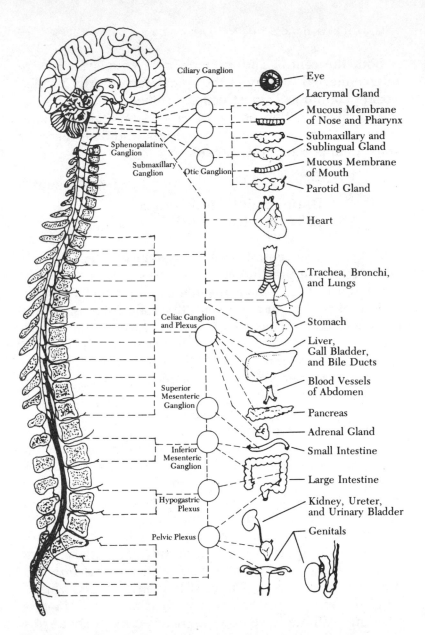

Figure 4–1. The nervous system, revealing two divisions: central and autonomic. From Schafer, **Chiropractic Health Care**. (Reprinted courtesy of The Foundation for Chiropractic Education and Research)

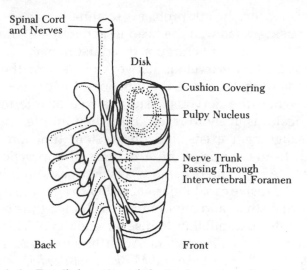

Spinal Cord
and Nerves

Disk

Cushion Covering

Pulpy Nucleus

Nerve Trunk
Passing Through
Intervertebral Foramen

Back

Front

Figure 4–2. Detailed section of the lumbar spine, showing the relationship between spinal nerves and spinal column.

Thirty-one pairs of nerves branch out from the spinal column. Each is made of millions of fibers less than one-hundredth the size of a human hair. Each nerve trunk passes through an opening called the *intervertebral foramen*, which is located between the vertebrae. This is the critical juncture where a misalignment can impinge on a nerve trunk and affect normal nerve transmission. In addition to the spinal nerves, our bodies contain twelve pairs of cranial nerves, which include the optic, acoustic, facial, and nasal nerves radiating to the eyes, ears, face, and nose (including the jaw), and the vagus nerve, passing through the neck and chest to the upper part of the abdomen.

Although cranial nerves work independently from spinal nerves, chiropractors take note of them for they, too, are affected by alterations in the blood supply. They receive transmissions from bundles of relay stations (known as *ganglia*) that are connected directly to the spinal nerves.

For this reason, health problems relating to ear, eye, and nasal passages (as well the head in general) are known to respond favorably to chiropractic adjustments. Through this marvelous network of nerves, the brain responds to and controls the function of every cell of the body. When the nervous system is free of interference, good health is likely to result. But when interference due to misalignment exists, nervous system function is impaired. In the words of the American Chiropractic Association, "An impaired nervous system may diminish the body's defensive capabilities, its ability to adapt to internal or external stress and environmental change thus contributing to its susceptibility to disease etiology." This belief is not limited to chiropractors. According to Dr. A. J. Cunningham in the text *Biological Mediators of Behavior and Disease*, disregulation of the central nervous system is increasingly being implicated as a contributing factor in disease, and can adversely affect the hormonal system, the immune system, and our general health.

The Spine: Your Pillar of Life

Long before Hippocrates, a healthy spine was recognized as vital to good health. Today, chiropractic is the only science specifically concerned with the proper care of the spine and the relationship between it and the nervous system.

The *spinal column*, the main shaft of the body, is composed of twenty-four movable bones called *vertebrae* (from the Latin word *vertere*, "to turn"). There are four principal groups of vertebrae (Figure 4–3). The seven most superior are the *cervical* vertebrae, which make up the neck. They are followed by twelve more in the upper or mid back known as the *thoracic* (or *dorsal*) vertebrae. The five below them are the *lumbar* vertebrae, the largest and heaviest

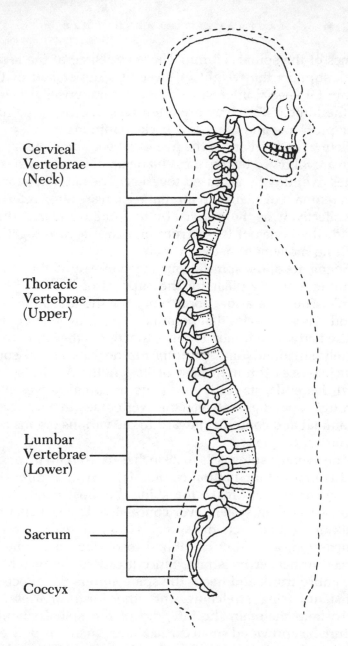

Cervical
Vertebrae
(Neck)

Thoracic
Vertebrae
(Upper)

Lumbar
Vertebrae
(Lower)

Sacrum

Coccyx

Figure 4–3. The spinal column. From Inglis, The Book of the Back.
(Reprinted courtesy of Ebury Press)

bones of the spinal column. These vertebrae of the lower back support the weight of the entire upper half of the body. Of special interest to chiropractors, misalignments of the lumbar vertebrae are often responsible for painful disc problems and other low back conditions.

Below the lumbar are the five *sacral* vertebrae, which in turn are followed by the *coccyx* made up of four (and sometimes five) tiny bones fused together. The latter appear to be a remnant of a tail, and for that reason are often referred to collectively as the *tailbone*. By the time we reach adulthood, the bones of the sacrum and coccyx fuse together with no movement between them.

Segments of the spine are arranged one upon the other, forming a strong pillar for the support of the head and trunk. They are also a focal point for the attachment of hundreds of muscles that permit the free movement of the entire body. In addition to these functions, the spine completely surrounds and protects the delicate spinal cord, which passes through most of its length. As the spinal cord descends, its thirty-one pairs of spinal nerves pass through openings between the vertebrae (intervertebral foramina) and continue onward to the various organs and tissues of the body.

The average spine is 24 to 28 inches (60–80 cm) in length and contains four natural *curves*, as seen in Figure 4–3. These curves help make the spine the most magnificent shock-absorbing system ever conceived. The fact that we walk upright subjects the spinal column to every kind of concussion, and from childhood to old age the spine is placed under terrific strain. Since it carries the weight of the entire trunk and head, the spine suffers the effects of constant jarring, stretching, and other forms of stress.

To help maintain the integrity of the spinal column, nature has provided small cartilaginous cushions between the vertebrae known as intervertebral discs. These discs are carefully fitted to give shape to the spine and to prevent excessive movement so that jarring and strain have minimal effect on the spine and nervous system. However, these spinal discs are constantly subject to gravity and torque from body movements and are therefore susceptible to wear and tear over the years. Spinal misalignments caused by falls, accidents, improper lifting, or sprains may allow the disc to "slip," bulge, herniate, or impinge upon a delicate spinal nerve (Figure 4–4). By realigning vertebral misalignments and subluxations, chiropractors relieve abnormal disc pressure. This has proven to be of benefit in relieving many so-called "slipped disc" conditions.

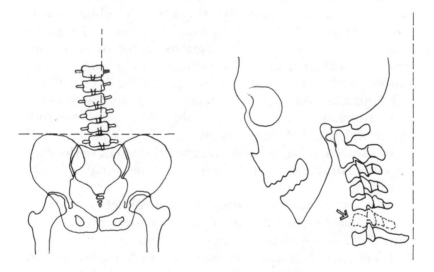

Figure 4–4. (Left) An abnormal curvature with several subluxations of the lower back. (Right) A subluxation of the sixth cervical vertebra. Note uneven disc space between vertebrae. From Schafer, Chiropractic Health Care. (Reprinted courtesy of The Foundation for Chiropractic Education and Research)

Subluxation: An Out-of-Line Response

The spine is so beautifully designed that the intervertebral foramina between the bones are exactly the correct shape and size to accommodate the big nerve trunks (along with veins and arteries) that pass through them. If the openings are properly maintained, nerve energy from the brain flows unimpeded through the nerve trunks and onward to eventually reach every cell of the body. But if one or more of the vertebrae are out of alignment, the opening becomes smaller as the result of a hard bone impinging on a soft nerve. A broad definition of subluxation was presented at a National Institute of Neurological and Communicative Disorders and Stroke (NINCDS) workshop on spinal manipulative therapy: "A subluxation is the alteration of the normal dynamics, anatomical or physiological relationships of contiguous [adjacent or adjoining] articular structures." In contrast, a definition recently approved by the Board of Directors of the International Chiropractors Association concerns itself more with nerve transmission: "The vertebral subluxation syndrome and/ or complex and its component parts is any alteration of the biomechanical and physiological dynamics of the contiguous structures which can cause neuronal disturbances."

Medical doctors often overlook the subtlety of subluxations, claiming that they are figments of the chiropractor's imagination. The fact that they exist and can have a powerful impact on health, however, has been documented in medical journals since 1909. The distinguished surgeon James P. Warbasse wrote: "Subluxations of the vertebrae occur in all parts of the spine and in all degrees. When the dislocation is so slight as not to affect the spinal cord, it will still produce disturbances in the spinal nerves, passing off through the spinal foramina."

Today, what is known scientifically as the *chiropractic*

subluxation complex or *CSC* is one of the most exciting areas of study in physical medicine. According to Robert Dishman, D.C., writing in the *Journal of Manipulative and Physiological Therapeutics*, "The 'chiropractic subluxation complex' may now be defined and described as a definitive clinical entity having broad and deep implications concerning pathogenesis." He added that the absence of the CSC "serves as a model for health and homeostasis by virtue of a normal neurobiomechanical system, the sine qua non of which is the vertebral column."

Disruption of the Nervous System: Some Case Histories

The relationship between the spine and the nervous system is extremely complex. Chiropractic research has determined that even the slightest misalignment can produce nerve interference that may surface with a variety of effects. According to Dr. Frank P. DeGiacomo of the New York Chiropractic College, "Anatomical disrelation either macroscopic or microscopic may disturb the normal generation, transmission, distribution, or expression of the nervous system, and may cause symptoms or pathology local to or remote from the particular region." This means that nerve interference may produce immediate or cumulative effects on any part of the body.

For example, an impinged nerve in the lower thoracic (midback) area may cause localized pain or weakness in an organ the nerve services, such as the colon. Constipation, spasticity, or colitis may result immediately or after a period of time. Impairment of the proper flow of energy through a nerve is usually followed by a malfunction in the organ that it serves.

Let's examine the case histories of two college athletes, Charles and Roy. Both were slightly injured during the football season and had similar subluxations in the thoracic areas of their spines. For Charles, the nerve impingement produced back pain, making it difficult to play on the team or even to attend classes. After several days of extreme discomfort, he sought out a local chiropractor who adjusted his spine, removing the cause of nerve interference. Within five minutes the pain was gone. The following Monday, Charles was back on the team.

Roy, in contrast, felt nothing and continued to play on the football team. Eighteen months later, however, he began to suffer from intestinal problems. (The intestine is one of the organs served by the impinged thoracic nerve.) Although the university health service gave medication to relieve chronic constipation and intestinal cramps, Roy's health did not improve. His teammate Charles suggested he visit his chiropractor. Roy received a series of chiropractic adjustments for several weeks (three per week for three weeks). The nerve supply to his intestinal organs was normalized and symptoms soon began to diminish.

A subluxation may be large enough to be recognized by the untrained eye or so small that it escapes the attention of all but the most experienced specialists. Recent studies have found that the degree of displacement has no direct correlation with the amount of nerve interference present. A tiny misalignment can inhibit the vital flow of cerebrospinal fluid for impulse transmission. Therefore, most chiropractors will pay attention to a tiny subluxation that the medical doctor or physical therapist may consider insignificant.

Regardless of the size of the subluxation, the resultant pressure on and possible irritation of the delicate spinal nerves may *increase* or *decrease* the flow of nerve energy to the organs or tissues served by the nerve. This can lead to dis-ease, which may, though not always, lead to actual physical symptoms. According to Dr. I. M. Korr, an osteopath who is an authority on both the osteopathic lesion and chiropractic subluxation: "The lesion/subluxation is a most important factor—it is a sensitizing factor, a localizing factor, a channeling factor. The lesion/subluxation sensitizes a segment of the cord, lowers the barrier, facilitates, without necessarily producing symptoms . . ."

How energy flow is affected depends on the particular individual's reaction. It cannot be determined in advance. The natural movements of the body correct most subluxations, but many go uncorrected for years. Although not immediately evident, an uncorrected misalignment can produce long-term effects that may result in permanent damage to nerves, organs, muscles, or to the spine itself, limiting movement and causing degeneration of vertebrae. When left uncorrected, a simple spinal misalignment can develop into a serious condition.

The sympathetic nervous system alone influences enzyme activity in the body, the regulation of DNA and RNA, the functions of the glands, circulation, the activity of bone cells, and basic growth and development. Although more research needs to be done concerning these and other functions of the nervous system and how they can be affected by nerve irritation or compression, much clinical and anecdotal information has been collected by researchers.

However, scientific studies also have documented a wide variety of problems that can be caused by vertebral subluxation. We mentioned earlier the findings of Dr. Abraham Towbin of Harvard, who found that severe subluxations have been associated with brain stem and cord injury that lead to hypoxia (lack of oxygen) and crib death (SIDS) among newborns, and of A. D. Speransky, a Soviet physician who found that damage to the spinal cord or nerve roots can result in pathological changes of lung tissue. In *The Research Status of Spinal Manipulative Therapy*, Dr. C. H. Suh, who headed the NINCDS study, found that "aberrant [unusual] neurological activity resulting from mechanical disorders of the spine is due to compression of spinal nerves at the intervertebral foramina." In an article in the *Journal of Manipulative and Physiological Therapeutics*, Scott Haldeman, who holds both D.C. and M.D. degrees, observed that "compression of a nerve interferes with the impulse transmission causing muscle paralysis, vasodilation, and trophic ulcers."

Compression of the spinal cord due to subluxations has also been linked with numbness and tingling of the hands and feet. Subluxations of the cervical vertebrae can compress the vertebral arteries, which can affect the blood supply to the head, producing manifestations such as headache, nausea, tinnitus, neuralgia, vomiting, dizziness, and "drop attacks." Restricted joint movement, abnormal muscular tone and texture, muscular tensions, postural problems, and limited and painful motions have also been clinically linked to vertebral subluxations.

Figure 4–5 is a simplified chart given out by chiropractors to patients. Although intended to show some of the possible effects of vertebral subluxations, the specific location of a subluxation does not necessarily lead to impaired function or illness in a specific area. Neurology is an extremely complex subject and the unique processes involving the spinal nerves and nerve transmission are far from fully understood. Therefore, reliable predictions cannot be made.

The Case of Henry

The following case history illustrates how an uncorrected subluxation can lead to a serious and complex state of ill health. Henry is fifty-two years old and owns a neighborhood stationery shop in a large midwestern city. Ten years ago, he suffered a major displacement in the midback when he took a bad fall on the ice while walking home from work. Although he felt severe pain for three weeks, he forgot about the incident as soon as the discomfort faded.

The subluxation involved the fifth thoracic spinal nerve leading to the liver and solar plexus.

Henry appeared to enjoy reasonably good health for years, but his liver had begun to malfunction in regulating the amount of cholesterol in the blood. Henry's love for hamburgers and sausages didn't help. It forced the liver to work that much harder purifying the blood of toxic bacteria, antibiotics, and hormones found in the meat. Henry felt heavy and bloated after a small meal and sometimes had to lie down while the liver slowly cleansed the blood.

Since the weakened organ was unable to function at peak efficiency, its ability to supply the brain with adequate amounts of oxygen and glucose (a sugar) was impaired. As a result, Henry often became irritable and had trouble sleeping. The liver's ability to store vitamins was also diminished, and the result was several vitamin deficiencies. By the time Henry was fifty years old, his cholesterol count and blood pressure had reached dangerous levels. He was a frequent visitor to his physician for tests and medical treatment, with mixed results.

By the time Henry finally consulted a chiropractor, he looked and felt twenty years older than his age and was a prime candidate for a heart attack or stroke. The chiropractor located the misalignment that was contributing to his trouble and adjusted it. After six weeks of care, which involved a chiropractic adjustment twice a week, he began to feel much better. Although not all body functions had returned to normal, his long-term chances for reclaiming health were good.

How Subluxations Occur

Subluxations are very common phenomena. We receive dozens of them every day. Although some cause pain, most do not and are beyond our awareness. The vast majority are corrected through normal spinal

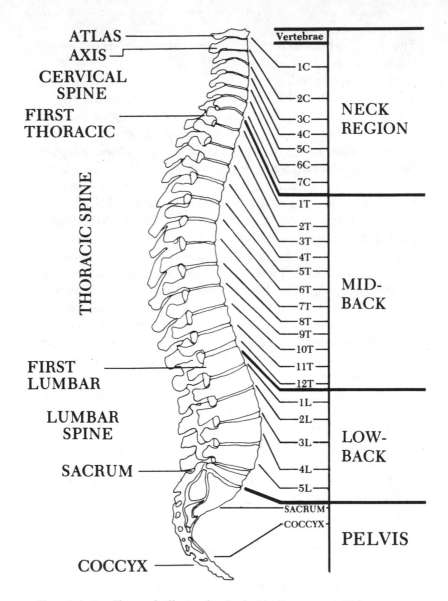

	Vertebrae	
ATLAS		
AXIS	1C	
CERVICAL SPINE	2C	NECK REGION
FIRST THORACIC	3C	
	4C	
	5C	
	6C	
	7C	
THORACIC SPINE	1T	
	2T	
	3T	
	4T	
	5T	
	6T	MID-BACK
	7T	
	8T	
	9T	
	10T	
FIRST LUMBAR	11T	
	12T	
LUMBAR SPINE	1L	
	2L	
	3L	LOW-BACK
SACRUM	4L	
	5L	
	SACRUM	
	COCCYX	PELVIS
COCCYX		

Figure 4–5. Chart of effects of spinal misalignments. "The nervous system controls and coordinates all organs and structures of the human body" (Gray's Anatomy, 29th ed., p. 4). *Misalignments of spinal vertebrae and discs may cause irritation to the nervous system and affect*

Areas	Effects
1C Blood supply to the head, pituitary gland, scalp, bones of the face, brain, inner and middle ear, sympathetic nervous system.	Headaches, nervousness, insomnia, head colds, high blood pressure, migraine headaches, nervous breakdowns, amnesia, chronic tiredness, dizziness.
2C Eyes, optic nerves, auditory nerves, sinuses, mastoid bones, tongue, forehead.	Sinus trouble, allergies, crossed eyes, deafness, eye troubles, earache, fainting spells, certain cases of blindness.
3C Cheeks, outer ear, face bones, teeth, trifacial nerve.	Neuralgia, neuritis, acne or pimples, eczema.
4C Nose, lips, mouth, eustachian tube.	Hay fever, catarrh, hearing loss, adenoids.
5C Vocal cords, neck glands, pharnyx.	Laryngitis, hoarseness, throat conditions such as sore throat or quinsy.
6C Neck muscles, shoulders, tonsils.	Stiff neck, pain in upper arm, tonsilitis, whooping cough, croup.
7C Thyroid gland, bursae in the shoulders, elbows.	Bursitis, colds, thyroid conditions.
1T Arms from elbows down, including hands, wrists, fingers; esophagus and trachea.	Asthma, cough, difficult breathing, shortness of breath, pain in lower arms and hands.
2T Heart, including its valves and covering; coronary arteries.	Functional heart conditions and certain chest conditions.
3T Lungs, bronchial tubes, chest, breast.	Bronchitis, pleurisy, pneumonia, congestion, influenza.
4T Gall bladder, common duct.	Gall bladder conditions, jaundice, shingles.
5T Liver, solar plexus, blood.	Liver conditions, fevers, low blood pressure, anemia, poor circulation, arthritis.
6T Stomach.	Stomach troubles, including nervous stomach; indigestion, heartburn, dyspepsia.
7T Pancreas, duodenum.	Ulcers, gastritis.
8T Spleen, diaphragm.	Hiccoughs, lowered resistance.
9T Adrenal and supra renal glands.	Allergies, hives.
10T Kidneys	Kidney troubles, hardening of the arteries, chronic tiredness, nephritis, pyelitis.
11T Kidneys, ureters.	Skin conditions such as acne, pimples, eczema, or boils.
12T Small intestines, lymph circulation.	Rheumatism, gas pains, certain types of sterility.
1L Large intestines, inguinal rings.	Constipation, colitis, dysentery, diarrhea, some ruptures or hernias.
2L Appendix, abdomen, upper leg.	Cramps, difficult breathing, acidosis, varicose veins.
3L Sex organs, uterus, bladder, knees.	Bladder troubles, menstrual troubles such as painful or irregular periods, miscarriages, bed wetting, impotency, change of life symptoms, many knee pains.
4L Prostate gland, muscles of the lower back, sciatic nerve.	Sciatica; lumbago; difficult, painful, or too frequent urination; backaches.
5L Lower legs, ankles, feet.	Poor circulation in the legs, swollen ankles, weak ankles and arches, cold feet, weakness in the legs, leg cramps.
SACRUM Hip bones, buttocks.	Sacro-iliac conditions, spinal curvatures.
COCCYX Rectum, anus.	Hemorrhoids (piles), pruritis (itching), pain at end of spine on sitting.

the structures, organs, and functions, which may result in the conditions shown above. (Reprinted courtesy of the Parker Chiropractic Research Foundation) movement when we stretch and move about during the day. When we sleep, spinal disc expansion occurs, and this too can correct minor subluxations.

According to Donald Epstein, D.C., subluxations are caused "by any stress . . . which our body cannot properly perceive, adapt [to] or recover from." Such stresses are primarily chemical, emotional, and physical in origin. By becoming aware of these causes, we can reduce the risk of subluxation, and consult a chiropractor if we do experience one of them.

Our Chemical Environment

After suffering an allergic reaction to an antibiotic, Diane felt mild back pain. Her chiropractor believed the subluxation he discovered after a spinal examination may have been due to the adverse drug reaction.

David just returned from a visit to Mexico, where the drinking water in a particular village made him ill. Although he wasn't aware of it, his body's reaction to the water brought about a vertebral misalignment.

John visits a chiropractor every two weeks, and his doctor always notices that he has an abnormally high number of subluxations to correct. He is certain that John's heavy cigarette smoking is the cause.

Daniel David Palmer was probably the first person to call attention to the importance of chemical irritants and toxins as major sources of spinal misalignments. Discussing them in his textbook, he wrote: "The poison, acting on certain nerves, irritates their structure. They in turn contract muscles which draw vertebrae out of alignment, thereby impinging upon nerves which go and affect certain portions of the body."

Fifty years later, a book written exclusively about spinal misalignments (*The Neurodynamics of the Vertebral Subluxation* by A. E. Homewood, D.C.) cited dozens of medical studies that substantiate Palmer's claim that solid, liquid, or gaseous toxins from food additives, tobacco, exhaust fumes, other environmental pollution, or drugs (legal and illegal) may cause nerves to react so that body structures, such as the muscles, can be affected enough to move a vertebra out of alignment. Although chiropractic cannot claim to eliminate the risk of environmental contamination, periodic adjustments can help mitigate the effects of living in a polluted environment.

Our Emotional Environment

Greg rushed to catch the 8 o'clock flight to Chicago. He gave himself plenty of time, but an accident on the freeway caused a mammoth traffic jam. After hectic driving on detours and side streets, he reached the boarding gate with only minutes to spare. As he collapsed exhaustedly into his seat, Greg realized that his head was pounding and his neck was stiff. The headache was gone by the time the plane touched down in Chicago, but the subluxation he suffered was not. After a month of low-grade neck pain and stiffness, Greg consulted a chiropractor who removed the pressure on a cervical nerve with a single painless adjustment.

If you have indigestion or suffer from toothache, the pain affects your mental state and may put you in a bad mood. By the same token, a state of mind can make you ill, as Greg's case illustrates. Medical science has documented that fear, rage, depression, and emotional shock can produce a variety of pathological conditions, including decreased immune system function, ulcer, heart problems, and stroke. Illnesses caused by mental or emotional stress are known as *psychosomatic* diseases.

Many chiropractors maintain that feelings can bring about subluxations. Similar to the body's reaction to chemical toxins, our posture can be altered by stress, which can set up a cycle of potentially harmful effects. For example, when we are fearful or angry, we tend to contract the shoulders and lower the head. This action, especially if extreme, causes increased tension, torque, or stretching of the nerve structures. This can, in turn, cause muscles to contract to move one or more vertebrae out of alignment as an adaptive measure.

In his work to integrate the human body with psychiatry, Wilhelm Reich, M.D., found that people retract the pelvic area in response to shame, fear, or anxiety about sex. The abnormal posture continued over a long period of time produces compensatory changes in body structure, which accent the primary and secondary curvatures of the spine. Dr. A. E. Homewood, former president of the Canadian Memorial Chiropractic College, wrote that chronic muscular tension may contribute to localized subluxations, which could become major if left uncorrected.

As stated in chapter 1, chiropractic is not a panacea for emotional disorders, but it can help us achieve a state of good mental health. By freeing our bodies of nerve interference, a major cause of internal stress is removed. As a result, a person is not only relieved of tension but can adapt more easily to stress and can function at a higher level of efficiency and emotional balance. By breaking the vicious circle of subluxation, pain, and emotional pressure, the chiropractor helps us enjoy a benign circle of vitality, adaptability, and emotional well-being.

The Physical Environment

Peter was standing in line waiting for tickets to a concert when he sneezed. Immediately he felt something "go out" in his back and could barely walk. After three chiropractic adjustments, Peter was able to walk again without pain.

Linda broke two ribs in a serious car accident. She also felt a tingling in her left leg, which the medical doctor believed was linked to spinal nerve trauma. After four months of chiropractic care, proper nerve transmission was restored to her leg and the tingling stopped.

George pulled some back muscles when he lifted a large box of tiles at work. The pain subsided after two days of heat treatments, but the subluxation wasn't detected until he saw a chiropractor for a routine visit three weeks later.

Millions of people suffer from subluxations related to chemical and emotional causes, but the case histories of misalignments due to physical trauma reflect the majority of patients who consult a chiropractor. Accidents, serious or minor, are the most common cause of subluxation. Slipping on the ice, falling off a bicycle or motorbike, or suffering from a whiplash injury in a car accident may result in a spinal misalignment impinging on a nerve. Shoveling snow, moving heavy furniture, and improper lifting (such as bending over to remove a sack of groceries from the trunk or back seat of a car) are also major causes of physical subluxation.

Many ordinary tasks performed during a normal working day place repeated and prolonged strain on the spine and connecting muscles. Dentists, for example, are constantly stooping to perform dental work on their patients. Taxi drivers and truckers spend most of their time sitting in unnatural positions in seats of poor orthopedic design that lack proper back support. Secretaries and writers spend much of their days sitting in a stooped position while working at word processors or typewriters. Auto mechanics and plumbers work in cramped, uncomfortable spaces. Farmers, carpenters, miners, athletes, dancers, and commercial artists work at jobs that produce stress and strain on the spine.

Of all occupations, however, homemaking is subject to the widest variety of hazards—lifting and carrying heavy packages and children, moving furniture, turning mattresses. Practically every job produces some unnatural strain on the spinal column, which can result in misalignment.

When we hear a small "click" or "pop" as we stretch,

a minor displacement is being corrected. But those of a more serious nature (caused by accidents, strains, strong emotional reactions, or toxins) are not easily corrected by the body and, therefore, call for the attention of a professional. According to the Commission of Inquiry into Chiropractic in New Zealand, chiropractors are the only health practitioners equipped by education and training to carry out the specialized task of removing nerve interference with chiropractic spinal adjustments.

However, there is general apprehension among prospective chiropractic patients. They do not really know what a chiropractor is or how he or she is educated and licensed. The following chapter will explain "what makes a chiropractor." It explores how the practitioner becomes uniquely qualified to perform the exacting process of analysis and adjustment and to be responsible for complete chiropractic care.

CHAPTER 5

The Education of the Chiropractor

Modern chiropractic colleges provide a high standard of specialized instruction not duplicated anywhere else. The regulations for chiropractic licensure in the United States and Canada define the limits of the chiropractor's domain. Throughout the world, professional organizations are working to maintain the highest level of competence within chiropractic. Let's see what this means to us as health consumers.

The Backbone of Chiropractic: Education

One of the greatest misconceptions people have about chiropractors concerns their education. Some believe that chiropractors take a substandard course of study at a medical school; others, who know that chiropractors attend special chiropractic colleges, believe that the schools are "diploma mills" that offer incomplete and unscientific courses of instruction. Let's trace the evolution of chiropractic education from its modest beginnings to the current specialized system of education of the highest caliber.

When Daniel David Palmer opened the Palmer Infirmary and Chiropractic Institute in 1897, the school had no entrance requirements and anyone who could afford the $450 tuition fee could enter. Its three-month curriculum offered courses in chiropractic philosophy and technique in addition to lectures in anatomy and physiology. Brief courses in pathology, sanitation, and recognition of symptoms were based on the *Family Medical Advisor*, a popular "do-it-yourself" health book of the day.

Because early chiropractic never set itself up to be a form of medical therapy, the education of chiropractors traditionally differed from that of medical doctors. Whereas medical schools devoted much of their time to teaching about symptoms, pathology, drug therapy, and surgery, chiropractic education stressed a thorough knowledge of the spine, nervous system, and the removal of nerve interference. Little attention was given to disease symptoms and pathology.

Since the early part of this century, organized medicine has been highly critical of chiropractic education, despite the fact that one-third of the graduates of the Palmer Institute in 1902 were also graduate physicians, surgeons, or homeopaths. Medical doctors pointed to their training as being superior and more scientific, and criticized early chiropractic colleges as diploma mills whose primary goal was to make money.

However, many forgot that high-quality medical education itself is a somewhat recent development and that many early medical schools were little more than fly-by-nights more concerned with making a fast profit than providing a sound medical education. Reports of early medical schools in the United States were so bad that the Carnegie Foundation commissioned Dr. Abraham Flexner, a respected educator, to evaluate the nation's medical schools. His report, issued in 1910, caused a furor among the public and the medical profession alike.

After making personal visits to 154 medical schools in the United States and Canada, Dr. Flexner concluded that only 31 of the schools deserved to exist. In describing the chemistry departments of the nation's medical schools, Flexner painted a grim picture:

It is indeed stretching terms to speak of laboratory teaching in connection with them at all. . . . The Mississippi Medical College, when visited, did not own a dollar's worth of apparatus of any description whatsoever. . . . At the Milwaukee Medical College, bacteriology is represented mainly by several wire baskets of dirty test tubes; Temple University [Philadelphia] has no individual outfit for students in any science at all. . . . At the University of Oregon [Portland] and Willamette [Salem, Oregon] there is no running water at the desks.

And what of the students' exams? In discussing the examination procedure at some of the Chicago medical schools (Chicago has long been the home of the American Medical Association), Flexner wrote:

They drop in as they please. . . . No technical questions were asked; the presumption is that the applicants won't remember details. Formerly, written examinations were used in part, but they were given up "because almost everybody failed." The most flagrantly commercial of the Chicago schools operate "pre-medical" classes, where a hasty cram, usually at night, suffices to meet the academic requirements of the Illinois state board.

Flexner's report generated such public concern that the majority of medical schools were closed down within a few years. During the following decades, the Rockefeller, Eastman, Rosenwald, and Harkness foundations contributed $200 million to upgrade those remaining. By 1965, the *Journal of the American Medical Association* reported that the last of the unqualified medical schools in the United States had finally closed its doors.

Because chiropractic was too young and obscure a profession to attract money from the large foundations, its leaders took it upon themselves to improve the level of chiropractic education and bring the nearly one hundred chiropractic colleges in existence closer to the level of the upgraded, modern medical schools. The Congress of Education was established in 1947 by what is now the American Chiropractic Association. When the results of a study showed that the majority of practitioners wanted to improve the standard of chiropractic education to a uniform level that would qualify their accrediting agency for Department of Health, Education, and Welfare approval, an ambitious campaign aimed at achieving high educational standards was launched by the chiropractic profession itself.

As a result, many colleges had to close their doors and merge with stronger chiropractic institutions. Today, many schools are the result of two or three such mergers. No large foundations, no drug companies, and no government agencies gave money toward chiropractic education, yet college standards improved dramatically. In August 1974, the Council of Chiropractic Education (CCE) was recognized by the U.S. Office of Education of the Department of Health, Education, and Welfare as a valid accrediting agency for chiropractic colleges.

At the time of this writing, all but three schools enjoy membership status with the CCE. The others have chosen to affiliate with the Straight Chiropractic Academic Standards Association (SCASA), an accrediting agency that they believe is more qualified to set standards for a more conservative chiropractic education. In August 1988, the new U.S. Department of Education granted national recognition to SCASA as a specialized accrediting agency for straight chiropractic colleges. A complete listing of chiropractic colleges can be found in Appendix I.

Chiropractic Education Today:
Curriculum Qualifications

In most U.S. states and Canadian provinces, students of chiropractic are required to have earned sixty college credits (approximately two years) with special emphasis on biology, physics, and chemistry before beginning advanced study in a chiropractic college. By the time they are qualified for graduation, they have taken a resident course of study and training totaling at least 4400 sixty-minute class hours. This represents four years of college covering a period of nine months each year.

The basic curriculum of chiropractic education is composed of many subjects. Basic science courses include anatomy, physiology, chemistry, pathology, bacteriology, nutrition, hygiene, sanitation, and public health. Clinical courses include physical, clinical, laboratory, and differential diagnosis; gynecology; obstetrics; pediatrics; orthopedics; roentgenology (X-ray); first aid; gerontology; dermatology; toxicology; psychology; principles and practice of chiropractic; spinal analysis; and adjustive techniques. Elective courses are offered in jurisprudence, ethics, and economics. Some schools may offer instruction in kinesiology, physical therapy, meridian therapy, and minor surgery. Some chiropractic colleges offer Bachelor of Science degrees, as well as postgraduate and continuing education programs. This comprehensive program offers the modern chiropractor a thorough grounding in the basic health sciences and enables him or her to provide the finest health care to the widest possible variety of patients.

The majority of college faculty hold Doctor of Chiropractic (D.C.) or Ph.D. degrees. The others with master's degrees are encouraged to seek advanced training in their area of expertise. Many faculty are graduates of the schools in which they teach, conducting courses such as technic (adjustment techniques), roentgenology, and philosophy that are primarily chiropractic in scope. During the past few years, however, colleges have been recruiting professors outside the profession to teach courses such as chemistry, microbiology, clinical nutrition, and psychology. In addition, many schools have made efforts to recruit chiropractic faculty from other institutions in order to avoid excessive inbreeding of their staffs.

For the most part, chiropractic colleges place more emphasis on anatomy and neurosciences and devote less attention to drug therapy, surgery, and epidemiology. Many courses required for graduation compare favorably with those taught in medical schools. Some are even taught by medical doctors. In areas of special interest such as clinical nutrition and public health, there are more hours of instruction in chiropractic colleges than in most medical schools. Table 5–1 compares graduation requirements for a medical school and a chiropractic college, both located in the eastern United States.

In order to graduate, students must intern about 900 hours in a college-operated clinic and pass either of two tests. Those who pass the National Board of Chiropractic Examiners exam are recognized by most state licensing boards and by the vast majority of the Basic Science Exam Boards. The National Board of Chiropractic Examiners exam stresses general anatomy, spinal anatomy, physiology, pathology, microbiology, chemistry, and public health. It also focuses on general diagnosis, neuromusculoskeletal diagnosis, X-ray, principles of chiropractic, chiropractic practice, and associated clinical sciences. There is also the Physiotherapy Examination and the Written Clinical Competency Examination (WCCE), which is designed to assess clinical competence and practice skills. The WCCE focuses on nine clinical areas: case history, physical examination, neuromusculoskeletal examination, roentgenologic (X-ray) examination, clinical laboratory and "special

Table 5–1. Comparison of course hours required
for graduation

Course	Medical School	Chiropractic College
Anatomy	296	800
Biology of Disease/Biometrics/Cell Biology	562	—[1]
Biochemistry	80	160
Endocrinology	40	(80)[2]
General Medicine	460	—
Chiropractic Technique and Philosophy	—	816
Microbiology	103	192
Neurosciences	120	(272)[3]
Obstetrics and Gynecology	220	160
Pathology	123	336
Pediatrics	220	32
Diagnosis	174 (physical)	480
Radiology	(15)[4]	240
Surgery	460	—
Pharmacology	126	—
Psychiatry/Psychology	249	64
Clinical Nutrition	—	96
Community Medicine/ Epidemiology	18	—
Public Health	—	176
Home-Medical Science	160	—
Socio-Medical Science	66	—
Office Procedure and Jurisprudence	—	32
Clinic	—	888
Electives and other required courses	1700 (incl. clinic)	288
Total Hours	5222	5112

[1]Similar course material offered in various departments
[2]Offered in Dept. of Pathology
[3]Offered in Depts. of Anatomy, Diagnosis, and Physiology
[4]Included with Anatomy, Cell Tissue Biology, and Physiology

studies" examination, diagnosis or clinical impression, chiropractic techniques, supportive techniques, and case management.

State Law: Rules and Regulations

All U.S. states and most Canadian provinces license chiropractors to adjust the spine and related structures such as the arms and legs and may permit the use of drugless adjuncts such as massage, hydrotherapy, physiotherapy, heat and cold therapies, exercise, acupressure, and nutritional therapy. However, each state has special regulations defining the nature of chiropractic and limiting the kinds of services provided. Some regulations, such as prohibiting the use of drugs and major surgery, were included at the initiative of the chiropractic profession itself. Others, such as limiting the use of X-rays, were passed at the insistence of organized medicine to limit competition.

In New York, for example, the use of chiropractic X-rays is limited to patients over eighteen years of age, and chiropractors are not allowed to treat cancer, heart trouble, diabetes, or communicable diseases. (However, chiropractors who do not claim to treat specific diseases are able to care for patients with any health problem.) A chiropractor in New York State may not take blood tests, but a chiropractor in Nevada may because all methods of diagnosis are permitted by Nevada state law. The use of prescription drugs or surgery is prohibited in every state except Oregon, which, according to the *Official Directory of Chiropractic and Basic Science Examining Boards*, allows the removal of warts and other "foreign bodies in the superficial structures and the use of antiseptics and local anesthetics in connection herewith." However, at the time of this writing, nonprescription proprietary drugs (such as aspirin and ibuprofin) may be administered in Florida, Vermont, Illinois, and Texas.

Regulations for soft tissue manipulation vary as well. Massage is permitted in California as long as it is performed in relation to spinal adjustments. Hawaiian law expressly prohibits chiropractors from performing the Hawaiian practice of "lomilomi or massage" as part of their profession. The myriad of state regulations cover even postmortem conditions. If a person dies of a heart attack or an accident in South Dakota, California, or Tennessee, a chiropractor may legally sign the death certificate, but not if the death occurs in Wisconsin, Massachusetts, Arizona, or twenty-one other states.

The Chiropractor's Domain: Adjustment or Referral

Even with years of specialized instruction and with strict licensing requirements on state and national levels, chiropractors find that some people still doubt their qualifications. These doubts can be expressed in the following two questions: (1) Doesn't a chiropractor treat too wide a range of disease? (2) Is a chiropractor qualified to recognize diseases that should receive the attention of a medical doctor?

The answer to the first question is no. *Chiropractic is not primarily a disease- or symptom-care system.* Although practitioners are taught diagnosis in college, symptoms are viewed primarily as guideposts in selecting the proper clinical procedure to eliminate nerve interference.

Chiropractors often address the issue of disease treatment by explaining the chiropractic view of the four phases of illness. Phase one is the *production of cause*, which may be interference with nerve transmission somewhere between the brain and one or more organs of the body. The second phase is *alteration of function*, or the failure of some organ or organs, with a resulting upset in the chemical balance of the body. Phase three includes *symptoms, signs, and syndromes*, which tell us we are not feeling well. The fourth phase is *actual structural change* involving the pathological degeneration of tissue in the affected body part.

In chiropractic, the production of cause is seen as primarily vertebral subluxation, which can impair the proper functioning of the nervous system. An impaired nervous system may diminish the body's defensive capabilities and its ability to adapt to internal or external stress. This can, in turn, weaken the body's ability to resist disease, which weakness may reveal itself in symptoms, signs, and syndromes. The medical doctor begins work by classifying and naming the effects of body dysfunction, otherwise known as *diagnosis*. Then he or she applies treatment to these advanced stages of illness.

The primary goal of the chiropractor, conversely, is not to diagnose symptoms (which implies distinguishing one disease from another), but to analyze a structural condition and decide how to correct it. This does not mean that a chiropractor ignores his or her extensive training in diagnosis. Through a complete and highly detailed case history, every aspect of the patient's physical, emotional, and mental situation is taken into account. However, unlike the physician, the diagnosis of disease is not the chiropractor's main goal. Chiropractic diagnosis primarily serves to determine the presence and character of a subluxation or related biomechanical problem.

If a patient has cancer, a heart condition, or any other disease, he or she is said to be a chiropractic case *as long as a vertebral subluxation exists*. This does not imply that a chiropractic case cannot be a medical case as well. Most people come to chiropractors only after their symptoms are severe. When a patient's condition requires allopathic treatment, it is a chiropractor's duty to refer him or her to the appropriate practitioner. During the past few years, chiropractors and medical doctors have begun to work together to provide the highest level of patient care.

The second question, regarding the ability of a chiropractor to recognize diseases that should receive medical attention, is closely related to the issue of referral. Although chiropractors do not receive the same amount of training in symptomatology as medical doctors, the New Zealand study concluded that "the education and training of a registered chiropractor are sufficient to enable him to determine whether there are contra-indications to spinal manual therapy in a particular case, and whether the patient should have medical care instead of or as well as chiropractic care."

Many chiropractic practitioners point out that the majority of their patients come to them after traditional medicine has failed and ailments are thoroughly documented. Ninety-seven percent refer clients to medical doctors and other specialists when they think these others can be the most help to the patient. Chiropractors do not claim to overly extend or limit their areas of expertise. They are bound by professional ethics to hold the welfare of their patients as their highest goal.

Quality Control:
The Professional Organizations

Currently, there are three national organizations whose role is to establish and maintain standards of education, ethics, and professional competency. They also represent the profession before the U.S. Congress and other government bodies. The larger organizations promote research programs, whereas all three disseminate information to their members and the general public. Many chiropractors are members of more than one professional organization, and an estimated one-third are not members of any.

The American Chiropractic Association (ACA) is the largest of the three. A successor to the National Chiropractic Association (NCA), which was founded in 1905, the ACA represents the majority of chiropractors in the United States and counts approximately half of all licensed chiropractors among its members. Its national headquarters is located just outside Washington, D.C., and includes state and local associations throughout the country. The ACA sponsors professional councils on mental health, neurology, orthopedics, diagnosis and internal disorders, diagnostic imaging, physiological therapeutics, nutrition, sports injuries and physical fitness, and technic. The ACA also supports chiropractic research and sponsors a variety of health education activities.

The International Chiropractors Association (ICA) was founded by B. J. Palmer in 1926 to represent the profession's conservatives. Located in suburban Washington, D.C., the ICA is composed of chiropractors throughout the United States and many foreign countries, and its Assembly is composed of elected members from each of the fifty states. In addition to promoting chiropractic research, high professional standards, and lobbying, the ICA, like the ACA, is involved with student recruitment and sponsors an active program of patient and public education.

The Federation of Straight Chiropractic Organizations (FSCO) was founded in 1976 by a group of extremely conservative chiropractors who believed that the ICA was too close to the liberal philosophy of the ACA and the Council of Chiropractic Education. Claiming a membership of over two thousand and made up of a house of delegates from each affiliate group, the FSCO endorses a strict code of professional ethics and the education of the public and other chiropractors in its "straight" philosophy. It is regarded as extreme by other chiropractic organizations.

Besides the three groups in the United States, professional organizations exist in most countries where chiropractic is officially recognized. The largest include organizations in Canada, Australia, and Great Britain. The European Chiropractors Union is composed of member organizations throughout the Continent. A complete listing of chiropractic professional organizations can be found in Appendix II.

All chiropractic organizations have a code of ethics and disciplinary procedures for their members. In the United States, each affiliate is similar to its parent organization. It has peer review guidelines implemented when a member's ethics or professional conduct is questioned on either state or local levels. In addition, the state-operated Division of Professional Licensing Services in each state is equipped to deal with complaints about unethical or incompetent practitioners, be they chiropractors, dentists, optometrists, or medical doctors. Over the years, the chiropractic profession has achieved the highest standards of educational and professional competence. Whether you need help for a physical ailment or preventive health care, you can be assured of the services of a trained professional well qualified to perform chiropractic's specialized tasks.

Although most practitioners agree on the essential philosophy of their profession—the need to correct nerve interference—the three national organizations in the United States highlight the different points of view in chiropractic philosophy and practice. In the following chapter we will examine these varying points of view to see how their different approaches can influence the kind of care we receive.

CHAPTER 6

Choosing the Right Chiropractor

According to statistics provided by the Federation of Chiropractic Licensing Boards, there are over forty thousand licensed chiropractors in the United States and Canada. At least one chiropractor can be found in even the smallest hamlet or farm community throughout English- and French-speaking North America. In rural areas, your choice may be limited to the only one in town, but if you live in a city or suburb you will want to choose a chiropractor who meets your personal needs best.

Like the seeking out of any health professional, the selection of a chiropractor should be a careful and thorough process. After locating the name of a chiropractor, find out his or her standing in the community. Decide whether this person's philosophy of health and disease is compatible with your own and decide if you want the services of a conservative "narrow scope" or a liberal "broad scope" chiropractor, or one in between. Find out which techniques will be used in your care. Many patients want to know the extent of the use of X-rays, and if they are required before care begins. Be sure to understand the financial requirements. Find out if long-term contracts are required before the chiropractor will begin giving adjustments. Finally, see how a chiropractor feels about promises of "miracle cures" and if patients are referred to other practitioners when necessary.

Finding before Choosing: Your Sources

The first logical step in choosing a chiropractor is to find one. This can be done by writing to one of the professional organizations listed in Appendix II, looking in a local newspaper or weekly advertiser, or using the Yellow Pages in a local phone book, which may list chiropractors according to the town or neighborhood in which they practice.

The most reliable way to find one is to ask friends, relatives, and neighbors. With one American in twenty visiting a chiropractor this year, chances are excellent that you know several patients already. Since the chiropractic profession is largely dependent on referrals, chiropractors make an effort to provide the highest possible level of care. Those who are incompetent or unethical or have difficult personalities will receive little community support. Many encourage patients to bring friends and relatives to witness the examination and adjustment procedure. Some sponsor free lectures to educate the public. Chiropractors believe the more they are observed in practice, the faster the myth portraying them as "quacks" and "bone crushers" will dissolve.

In many ways, the chiropractic profession is like a big family. Personal and professional ties established in college and at seminars are often maintained for life. If you are a patient already but expect to move to another community, your current chiropractor can often recommend several others who share the same philosophy or technique you are accustomed to. If you want chiropractic maintenance care during a journey, your practitioner may be able to provide a set of X-rays and written observations along with a list of recommended professionals to consult on your trip.

Your Choice: Broad- or Narrow-Scope Care

Many patients choose a chiropractor for a particular philosophy and range of services rather than for personality or standing in the community. As pointed out in chapter 3, most chiropractors agree on the basic principles as taught by Daniel David Palmer, but differ on secondary considerations regarding the scope and practice of their profession. Although all licensed chiropractors are qualified to locate, analyze, and remove subluxations of the spine, their various attitudes toward health care play a major role in the type of care we receive. These beliefs and goals are often confusing to the prospective chiropractic patient, and I will attempt to clarify them here.

The conflict involves conservative chiropractors with a narrow scope of practice (known as "straights") and liberal chiropractors with a broad scope of philosophy and practice (branded as "mixers" by D. D. Palmer). Conservatives claim that their role does not involve the diagnosis or treatment of disease but involves the analysis and correction of spinal subluxations for the removal of nerve interference only. Dr. Virgil V. Strang, Dean of Philosophy and Director of Professional Ethics at Palmer College of Chiropractic, spoke of this unique task when he wrote: "The chiropractor offers one service—only one—which is not duplicated by any other branch of the healing arts. That most distinctive, valuable, and potent service is the detection and removal of subluxations which are causing abnormal functioning of the nervous system."

Broad-scope chiropractors agree that although their major task may be the restoration of nerve transmission through the removal of subluxations, they should, as primary-care practitioners, be concerned with other causes of ill health and disease pathology. In addition to believing that chiropractic includes the diagnosis of disease, they advocate the use of adjuncts such as acupressure, nutritional therapy, electrotherapy, and physical therapy as safe and natural forms of treatment. According to Dr. G. Allen Stevens, in a letter to *The Chiropractic Journal*, "I believe in treating more than subluxations. I believe in using everything I can under the law to treat the patients who are under my care."

As can be expected, there is a wide range of belief and practice among chiropractors. For example, a narrow-scope chiropractor may lightly massage a patient's neck before giving an adjustment or suggest that the patient cut down on smoking. He could be accused of "mixing" by his more conservative colleagues, because such practices go beyond the detection, analysis, and removal of subluxations only.

Most people are unaware of the controversies within the chiropractic profession, which prefers to keep its differences "within the family." However, as the chiropractic profession plans to celebrate its centennial, many within it fear that it could actually separate into two basic camps. Not only would this divide and weaken the chiropractic profession in the long term, but it would affect its legal status, the education requirements of chiropractic students, licensure for graduates, and its continued inclusion in Medicare, Medicaid, and commercial insurance policies. For this reason, any conflicts within the profession can have a profound effect on the kind of health care available to us as health-care consumers. To the extent that such differences are left unresolved by the chiropractic profession, the public suffers.

A Contrasting View of Health and Disease

The cause of ill health is a major part of the philosophical differences among chiropractors. Although chiropractors agree that a healthy nervous system is of primary importance for the maintenance and recovery of health, some early practitioners did not agree with D. D. Palmer's contention that 95 percent of all disease is caused (directly or indirectly) by spinal subluxations. They believed, as most do today, that mental attitude, environment, heredity, and nutrition play major roles in determining health and resistance to illness. This led them to an interest in other aspects of disease. The vertebral subluxation was regarded as just one factor of many.

Defenders of Palmer's conservative approach do not discount the importance of the factors listed above, but they point out that pollution, poor diet, and a poor emotional state do their greatest damage by causing subluxations that in turn cause nerve interference and thence ill health. Noting that spinal misalignments and resultant nerve interference form a major threat to the body's ability to adapt to stress, defend itself from germs, maintain homeostasis, and heal itself, they feel that the correction of subluxations is their primary goal as specialists in chiropractic. They say, "Leave other aspects of health care to other specialists, such as nutritionists, osteopaths, and acupuncturists."

The two approaches result in different goals. Conservative chiropractors are primarily interested in locating, analyzing, and correcting vertebral subluxations with the intent to eliminate nerve interference, which they believe is the primary cause of dis-ease. They feel that as long as there is *no interference* to normal nerve function, inner wisdom will heal the body as it sees fit. Although they agree that many disease states have been known to respond to chiropractic adjustments, they claim it is an indirect result of the removal of nerve interference rather than a therapeutic procedure as such.

Liberal or broad-scope chiropractors believe that correcting nerve interference is only part of their holistic approach to health. According to the Master Plan of the American Chiropractic Association, which promotes a liberal philosophy, "Chiropractic is a branch of the healing arts which is concerned with human health and disease processes." It also states that the practices and procedures employed by chiropractors can include not only adjustment and manipulation but first aid, hygiene, sanitation, rehabilitation, and physiological therapeutic procedures "designed to assist in the restoration and maintenance of neurological integrity and homeostatic balance." In addition to traditional chiropractic analysis techniques, broad-scope chiropractors often utilize blood tests, urinalysis, electrocardiograms, and muscle testing (applied kinesiology) to determine the nature and extent of the health complaint. As mentioned earlier, adjunctive therapies often include acupressure, physical therapy, massage, galvanic current, and ultrasound. Their goal is to provide the widest range of natural services to their patients, and they see no conflict in offering drugless therapies in addition to chiropractic adjustments.

Each individual state has legislated the range of services that a chiropractor may legally provide. Some limit the chiropractor to adjustments of the spine and related articulations, such as the arms and legs. Others license chiropractors to peform minor surgery and prescribe and sell proprietary drugs like aspirin and ibuprofin.

Diagnosis versus Analysis

The whole issue of "the diagnosis and treatment of disease" is a major source of conflict within the profession. Broad-scope chiropractors use both terms, whereas narrow-scope straights take pains to use the words *analysis* and *adjustment*.

Liberal chiropractors point out that the term *diagnosis* has several meanings. One definition states it involves the art of recognizing a disease by its symptoms through examination of body fluids, secretions, and excretions, or by measuring heartbeat, blood pressure, and body temperature. Along with medical doctors, many broad-scope chiropractors use such indicators to determine the nature and degree of pathology and then offer the appropriate therapy or therapies to relieve it. Another meaning that refers to physical diagnosis involves the use of inspection, palpation, X-ray, or other methods to identify deviations from the normal (such as spinal misalignments). Because a chiropractor is considered a "primary health-care provider" by the government, liberal chiropractors claim that physical diagnosis (even in the medical sense) is necessary and, therefore, that the term *diagnosis* should be used within the profession.

Although acknowledging the importance of a well-rounded scientific background, conservatives believe that diagnosis in the medical sense is beyond the scope of chiropractic except when referring a patient to a medical doctor. Because conservative chiropractors from D. D. Palmer onward have sought to keep their profession a separate and distinct healing art from allopathic medicine, they balk at using terms such as *diagnosis* that are generally identified with medical practice. They see their role as performing chiropractic spinal *analysis*, meaning "an examination of anything (such as the spinal column) to distinguish its component parts or elements, separately or in relation to the whole." Because a vertebral subluxation cannot be diagnosed in the medical sense, they feel that the term *analysis* should be used. They also point out that the phrase "primary health-care provider" simply denotes an independent practitioner (such as a dentist or podiatrist) whose services can be rendered without a prescription from someone else—it does not necessarily call for the diagnosis of symptoms.

Finally, conservatives argue that if chiropractors claim to diagnose disease, organized medicine will have a foolproof case for its setting standards of chiropractic education, because diagnosis is a medical specialty. Since medical doctors are trained extensively in diagnosis and symptomatology, chiropractors who want to compete with them should go to a medical school or osteopathic college and specialize in manipulative therapy. Many chiropractic colleges now offer courses in medical diagnosis that compare favorably to those offered in some medical schools.

Treatment versus Adjustment

Let's imagine that you are in a chiropractor's office complaining of constipation. After assessing your condition, the broad-scope chiropractor would outline a detailed program of treatment to alleviate the symptoms and keep them from returning. In addition to chiropractic adjustments, which may or may not continue after symptoms disappear, your practitioner may recommend a high-fiber diet, colonic irrigation, and the use of herbal teas. If blood tests reveal certain deficiencies, a variety of vitamin and mineral supplements would be recommended (and often offered for sale) by the chiropractor.

In contrast, after the narrow-scope chiropractor determines that you suffer from a vertebral subluxation, a series of adjustments would be given along with a recommended program of preventive chiropractic care to continue after disease symptoms disappear. You might be told that the goal was not to relieve constipation, but that it would probably disappear when the body's normal nerve transmission is restored to normal. If the chiropractor thought that you may have a vitamin deficiency or were not eating properly, he or she might refer you to a certified dietitian, because providing dietary advice or nutritional supplements is not within the straight chiropractor's area of expertise.

Conservative chiropractors believe that the words *treatment* and *therapy* imply disease care, so they prefer not to use them. They echo D. D. Palmer's emphatic belief (though hopefully expressed in nonsexist terms) that chiropractic was never intended to stimulate or inhibit body functions through any kind of treatment or therapy, natural or unnatural:

> Chiropractic has no room for Miss Treatment, neither has adjustment any need of being hampered by Miss Remedy. These girls of fashion change their clothing to suit every suitor. . . .
> Chiropractors are not therapeutists. The chiropractic science is not therapeutical. A chiropractor repairs by adjusting, fixing, replacing [vertebrae]; he does not use any therapeutical remedies. Chiropractic is nontherapeutical.

For this reason, chiropractors use the term *adjustment* or *correction* (as in "correcting a subluxation"), which does not imply the treatment or cure of pathology or disease state.

Choosing: The Pros and Cons

Extremes of conservative and liberal philosophies can be a source of confusion, particularly when it comes to choosing the kind of care you want for yourself and your family. Despite the tendency to see one side as right and the other as wrong, both aspects have their positive "keynote qualities" as well as distortions. By sifting through the pros and cons, you can appreciate the essence of their contrasts and choose the type of care you think will meet your needs.

The positive quality of conservatives is an abiding respect for the inborn intelligence of the body and a deep confidence in its ability to heal itself. If you complained of asthma, for example, the practitioner would primarily look for a vertebral subluxation and adjust it. Although aware of any contraindication to chiropractic adjustments (such as spinal tumors or a fractured vertebra) and able to recognize situations that could be referred to a different type of practitioner, he or she would locate, analyze, and adjust the subluxation, trusting that after normal nerve transmission was restored, the body would heal itself from the inside out.

For the most part, conservative chiropractors do not involve themselves with therapeutic approaches that may be beneficial to the patient. If you had chronic constipation and were in need of immediate relief, enemas, herbs, or diet therapy would not be recommended, because the narrow-scope chiropractor is not involved in the treatment of disease. This can be frustrating for the patient who is looking for relief of uncomfortable or painful symptoms.

Ultraconservatives claim it is not their concern as chiropractors if you are forty pounds overweight, smoke a pack of cigarettes a day, and eat junk food at every meal. They don't even show you how to prevent subluxations. This doesn't mean that they don't care. They feel that their specialty is the analysis and removal of subluxations, which will help your body deal with these issues as its innate intelligence is able to express itself through a nervous system free of interference. As innate intelligence is able to express itself, conservatives claim that you will naturally seek out better diets, undertake proper exercise, and do whatever else is best for you. They maintain that matters of life-style, stress management, and nutrition should be referred to other professionals in their own areas of expertise. Such an attitude may annoy patients who want their chiropractors to provide them with a broad range of services as opposed to only one.

Perhaps the best quality of broad-scope chiropractors is their openness to new health trends and their interest in integrating several approaches to health in their work. They often possess a sincere desire to remove pain and to help the patient overcome disease using whatever natural, noninvasive methods are at their disposal. For example, in addition to a chiropractic adjustment, a visit with Dr. Randolph Meltzer may include electrical stimulation of acupressure points to restore body balance, a complete reflexology treatment, nutritional counseling, a session of sound and color therapy, and a massage. According to *Whole Life Times*, Dr. Meltzer believes that "ultimately, the purpose of all these therapies is to balance a person at all levels at once, structurally, nutritionally, and energetically."

Liberal chiropractors cite that chiropractic should not be as narrow as the Palmers or their followers have proposed. They point out that Dr. Solon Langworthy, a student of D. D. Palmer who later opened a chiropractic school in Cedar Rapids, Iowa, introduced massage and other adjuncts to chiropractic in the early part of this century. They also correctly point out that a broad-scope chiropractor is often the only practitioner who provides a wide range of holistic health-care options, thus fulfilling an important need in the community. Many practitioners have other specialists on staff in order to provide a variety of adjunctive therapies.

The negative aspect of the liberal approach is not unlike an attitude of some medical doctors: "I can do anything." In offering a wide variety of therapies to "fix up" the patient, the chiropractor uses educated intelligence to inhibit or stimulate body functions, a method common in medical practice. Their critics, conservative practitioners such as Dr. Fred H. Barge, feel that chiropractors who engage in what he calls "medipractice" should become osteopaths or change their title to "holiopaths." Philosophy aside, others claim that the use of adjuncts often can justify a higher fee, a concern to patients who are not covered by health insurance.

All things considered, the controversy between the narrow-scope straights and the broad-scope mixers has positive aspects, and the consumer is the beneficiary. The wide range of philosophical differences within the profession offers a broad spectrum of quality health care for a variety of patient needs. If you want a form of safe and effective drugless therapy for treatment of a particular disorder, you might consider a broad-scope chiropractor, who is eminently qualified to diagnose and treat a wide range of disorders. However, if you want health care to keep your body free from nerve interference and indirectly remove symptoms, you would tend to seek the care of a conservative.

The tenets of each philosophy are proclaimed by professional groups such as the American Chiropractic Association and the Federation of Straight Chiropractic Organizations, but the vast majority of chiropractors stand between the extremes. My own experience over a twenty-year period has led me to believe that classifications such as *straight* or *mixer, liberal* or *conservative, and broad-scope* or *narrow-scope* are arbitrary classifications that do not always reveal the true value of a chiropractor.

My first encounter was with an Illinois chiropractor after I injured my back by carelessly lifting a typewriter. The adjustment was for emergency purposes only. Our intent was to relieve painful symptoms as quickly as possible. When they were removed, I never returned to him again. My second experience was also with a treatment-oriented chiropractor, who gave me five chiropractic/acupressure sessions during the course of one week. He "fixed me up" by the end of the week as promised, and symptoms of fatigue, stress, and eye inflammation were relieved. Later experiences were with more conservative practitioners, who clearly stated that their goal as chiropractors was to remove nerve interference only. I have been very satisfied with their care.

In the preparation for this book, I have met dozens of chiropractors and patients. Although I am concerned about the growing trend of "more chiropractors and less chiropractic," I have come to the conclusion that regardless of philosophical belief, overall intent is of far more value to the patient than whether the chiropractor is liberal or conservative. Is the chiropractor more interested in service, or is money the principal factor? Does he or she encourage self-reliance, or encourage dependency? Are adjuncts used to satisfy genuine patient needs or are they included to increase the fee? Are X-rays absolutely necessary, or are they used to justify a higher fee? Is the chiropractor compassionate, taking the time to listen to the patient? Does the chiropractor reflect good health in his or her personal life, or is health just a theory to talk about? Whether we agree with conservatives or liberals, answers to the preceding questions will help us select the right chiropractor for our particular needs.

I mentioned before that it is important to discover if a practitioner's approach to health is compatible with your needs. You should question potential chiropractors about their philosophy and techniques. However, since many chiropractors advertise in local telephone directories and newspapers, their advertisements often reveal the kind of practice they maintain. There are no hard-and-fast rules, but the following key words in an advertisement will reveal the basic orientation:

Liberal broad-scope. Holistic health care; comprehensive chiropractic health care; adjunctive therapy; diagnosis and treatment for back pain (headache, sciatica, and so on); acupressure; applied kinesiology; massage; physiotherapy; acupuncture; traction; nutritional therapy or counseling; vitamin therapy; chiropractic physician; ACA member.

Conservative narrow-scope. None of the terms above, but may include the phrase "removal of nerve interference as a cause of" back pain (headache, sciatica, and so on); preventive chiropractic care; restoration of nerve function;

correction of vertebral subluxations; straight chiropractor; family chiropractor; ICA member; FSCO member.

X-Rays: Sometimes, Always, or Never

Most chiropractors take X-rays at one time or another as part of the regular examination. The use of X-rays, however, varies considerably. Some chiropractors use them rarely, limiting radiation to specific areas of the spinal column, but others frequently use full-spine X-rays that photograph from the base of the skull to below the pelvis to get an idea of how the entire spine is affected by vertebral subluxations.

Although many patients feel uncomfortable about being exposed to radiation, an X-ray will help determine if any contraindications to chiropractic care exist. For example, a hairline fracture of the second cervical vertebra may escape the scrutiny of a chiropractor during the initial examination. If an adjustment were given, there would be a chance that the vertebra would break apart and injure a delicate vein or artery. Roentgenograms also give a better understanding of the nature and extent of the vertebral subluxation, and enable the practitioner to make a more exacting adjustment. It's important to remember that the chiropractor receives more training in X-ray than the dentist, osteopath, or medical doctor, and is thoroughly qualified to know when X-rays are needed and how they can be obtained with minimum risk to the patient.

If you have never been to a chiropractor before, or are seeing one as a result of an accident, spinal X-rays are generally a good idea and can lead to better care. If you are concerned about radiation risk, ask for smaller X-rays focusing on specific areas of the spine. If it is advised that you have follow-up roentgenograms several months later, be satisfied they are necessary and not just a routine procedure. If you move to another community and plan to see a chiropractor there, ask for your current X-rays. They may not reflect the condition of your spine at the moment, but your next chiropractor will have a better idea of your major problems.

Some practitioners have a "waiver of X-rays" form for patients who refuse them. The waiver, signed by the patient, supposedly releases the chiropractor from responsibility if any "untoward effects develop or any further illness or injury develops directly or indirectly" as a result of treatment given without a complete chiropractic examination (to include X-rays, presumably) as recommended. These are used to encourage patients to accept X-rays, but some opt to sign it nevertheless and assume full legal responsibility for their care. If you are concerned about the dangers of frequent radiation, you may want to select a chiropractor who does not require X-rays as a prerequisite for care. Also, reject any practitioner advertising free X-rays. Radiation should never be used as a lure.

Techniques: All Safe, All Effective

Since all adjustive techniques correct subluxations safely and effectively, selecting a chiropractor who uses a particular style is basically a matter of preference. There are several dozen adjustment techniques in common use today. Some (such as Toftness and sacro-occipital technique) are so light that you can hardly feel them. Others, such as Palmer's "hole-in-one" featuring a dynamic thrust and rapid recoil, are more dynamic.

Many chiropractors utilize a variety of adjustment techniques and choose a specific one according to the type and location of the specific subluxation. Some chiropractors include light massage as a relaxing adjunct to adjustment. Others may play quiet music to help the patient relax. It is rare to find two chiropractors with identical methods and office procedures. Whatever the technique, chiropractic adjustments are safe, painless, and effective, *as long as they are administered by a licensed chiropractor.* (I'll describe the major chiropractic techniques in more detail in a later chapter.)

However, the final consideration of technique springs from the essential foundation of chiropractic: adjustment by hand. The majority of practitioners adhere to this fundamental concept, but some use mechanical devices to perform spinal corrections. Earlier models resembled an old-fashioned drill press, but modern instruments such as the Activator are small handheld devices designed to give a precise light-force adjusting thrust. Although such instruments appear to be popular with some recent graduates, most chiropractors believe that the safest, most effective way to make adjustments is by hand only.

The Payment Schedule: Know the Cost

The question of payments can be important, although some do not feel it is a major factor in choosing a chiropractor. Most chiropractors have a flat office fee payable by cash, check, or credit card at the conclusion of each visit. Discounts for ten or twelve adjustments paid in advance may be offered to encourage the patient to return for a predetermined number of visits within an alloted period of time. Besides the financial advantage of such a plan, regularity is important in successful chiropractic care. Advance payment may encourage the patient to keep appointments and continue adjustments, even after the initial symptoms disappear.

Before you decide, discuss finances with the practitioner and work out a payment schedule comfortable to both. Remember that restorative chiropractic care is often covered by Medicare and Medicaid in many states and most private insurance companies include chiropractic in their health-insurance policies. Your chiropractor knows if you are eligible for such insurance coverage and will provide the appropriate forms to help you make claims.

Rates vary widely but are usually half the regular office fee for a medical doctor in general practice. In 1990, the initial examination and consultation usually begins at fifty dollars and increases depending on the number of X-rays and other tests performed. The range of care is an important cost factor. A simple adjustment by a conservative practitioner, for example, may require five to ten minutes of office time and might cost from fifteen to twenty-five dollars. In contrast, a chiropractor who uses a variety of supplementary therapies would probably spend twenty to forty minutes with each patient and thus charge considerably more.

Other cost factors are determined by the chiropractor as an individual. One chiropractor I know of charges a set fee if you want to be adjusted immediately, but he gives a 50 percent discount if you don't mind waiting in line. A chiropractor specializing in family care has one fee for an individual but will adjust an entire family for only twice as much, even if the family includes ten children. One chiropractor has no set fees at all and suggests that patients pay what they can to the receptionist as they leave. A chiropractor located in a high-rent district in a large city will probably charge more than one whose office is located in a small farm community. It may be difficult to evaluate a chiropractor by the fee, but comparative shopping will help you find chiropractic care at the lowest possible price.

Notes of Caution

Promises, Promises

Chiropractic is an original approach because it was designed primarily as a health-care system rather than a disease-care system. It claims that spinal adjustments correct subluxations, which in turn helps restore the nervous system to greater efficiency, and that as nerve interference is removed a state of health is more likely to be present. Therefore, it is important to avoid chiropractors who promise complete cures in advertisements or in person, even if they cite cases similar to yours that have responded to chiropractic adjustments.

Contracts

Beware of any chiropractor (or any practitioner for that matter) who asks you to sign a contract for services. A written agreement is not a customary practice and you should consider very carefully before signing one. Very few patients have been victimized by licensed chiropractors, but if a contract is offered as a prerequisite for chiropractic care, seek legal counsel before you sign, or simply find another chiropractor.

Referrals

It is important to find a practitioner (whether a chiropractor or not) who is willing to refer you when another practitioner can do the most good. Over 95 percent of all chiropractors make referrals, so if your doctor does not refer patients—or maligns other practitioners or health-care professionals—you may want to find someone else. A degree of open-mindedness and respect for the basic good intent of other practitioners despite philosophical differences is the mark of a mature and sensitive doctor worthy of your attention.

CHAPTER 7

A Visit to a Chiropractor: What to Expect

Many people hesitate to consult a chiropractor. Aside from fears of doctors in general, some are not sure if their problems lie within the scope of chiropractic. Others fear that the chiropractic examination and adjustment may be a painful and even dangerous experience. Many prospective patients also are wary about the chiropractor's expertise and wonder if he or she is truly qualified to work with such a sensitive and complex structure as the spine.

The reality of a chiropractic visit is very different. New patients find that a chiropractor is a highly trained specialist who is concerned with their total health, rather than merely one body part or symptom. They also discover that a visit is neither painful nor dangerous. Many even find it a pleasurable experience. Let's explore the case of Kenneth Morrison, who is typical of many chiropractic patients.

Kenneth is a thirty-two-year-old house painter. Although his general health appeared satisfactory, he often complained of neck pain and occasional headaches. One of his coworkers suggested that Dr. Roberts, a local chiropractor, might be able to help him. Ken set up an appointment for the following Thursday after work.

When he entered the chiropractor's waiting room, Ken noticed with surprise how healthy the other patients looked. After receiving a warm welcome from the receptionist, he was given a case history to fill out. Although the form was similar to those used by medical doctors, it went into specifics about musculoskeletal complaints and asked him to make note of any fall, sprain, or accident he could recall. He was also surprised to find a question asking if his birth involved any complications or a cesarean section. Although Ken had a good safety record on the job, he remembered that at seventeen he was involved in a minor car accident. His head bumped against the windshield, which shattered. Although he had suffered only a few scratches and a headache, Ken's father took him to the hospital emergency room, where he was examined and sent home with a clean bill of health. Until he saw the case history form, Ken hadn't given the accident a second thought.

Consultation and Exam

By the time Ken completed the form, Dr. Roberts was ready to see him. The chiropractor's adjusting room looked more like a living room than a clinical office. It was free of the antiseptic odors, sterilizers, and needles often found at a medical doctor's. A large adjusting table stood at the center of the room and a model spine lay on the doctor's desk along with some framed photographs of his family. Several diplomas and charts were mounted on the walls.

When Ken discussed his case with the chiropractor, he was pleased to discover that Dr. Roberts took a personal interest in him and asked him about himself, not just his symptoms. Even though both knew that others were waiting outside for a consultation, Dr. Roberts didn't seem hurried, and he discussed the problem slowly in language that Ken could understand. Using the model spine as an example, he showed how vertebrae could become misaligned and impinge on spinal nerves. With the aid of a chart depicting the distribution of nerves throughout the body, Dr. Roberts showed how nerve interference in one part of the body can alter the function of an organ or tissue in another part. "Even a childhood fall from a bicycle can cause a spinal misalignment that can impinge on a nerve," he said. "You may not feel the effects for a long period of time. I think your car accident fifteen years ago may have been the beginning of your neck problem."

Dr. Roberts's attitude is typical among chiropractors. According to a 1974 survey by the University of Utah College of Medicine, chiropractors generated more patient satisfaction than medical doctors. Patients rated chiropractors especially high in personality and their ability to explain the problem and its care.

After the initial exchange of information, both were ready for the examination. The doctor asked Ken to remove his shirt and lie face down on the adjusting table, which was heavily padded and fitted with a special notch to cradle his head (Figure 7–1). Dr. Roberts then proceeded to examine Ken's back by hand, carefully palpating (examining by touch) each vertebra for any tenderness or bumps. He asked Ken "Does it hurt here?" when he found a tender area, and recorded his findings. Special attention was paid to the neck (or cervical) region. The second cervical vertebra (or axis) appeared to be out of alignment. The lengths of Ken's legs were compared (one was one-quarter inch shorter than the other), and the pelvis was found to be slightly askew. Dr. Roberts then had Ken stand up and bend to the left, the right, forward, and back. Using a plumb line to determine overall spine alignment, he found that Ken's left shoulder was slightly lower than the right and that his head tilted a bit to the left.

After this postural analysis, Ken sat on the table while his skin temperature was measured by a device called a *thermeter* (shown in Figure 7–2), a modern successor to the neurocalometer introduced by B. J. Palmer in 1925. Starting from the base of the skull, the doctor carefully moved the

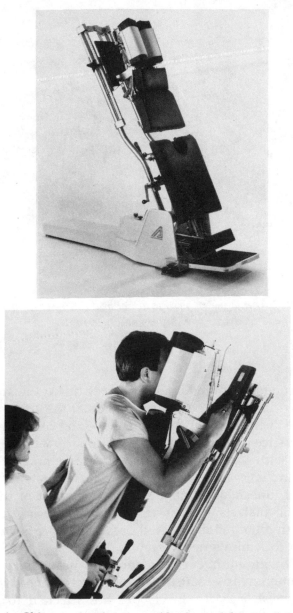

Figure 7–1. Chiropractic adjusting table, in upright and descending positions. (Courtesy of Williams Manufacturing)

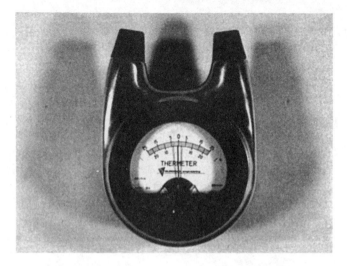

Figure 7–2. A thermeter, used to detect heat differentials on either side of the spine. (Courtesy of Murdoch Engineering)

two-pronged handheld device slowly down the spine, recording differences between one side of the spine and the other. When the temperature is lower on one side, nerve interference may be indicated. Dr. Roberts found four vertebrae with temperature differences and noted their location in Ken's chart. Other chiropractors sometimes include applied kinesiology (muscle testing) as part of their chiropractic analysis. By testing certain muscles of the body, they can often tell if a related organ or tissue is weak and trace it to a misaligned vertebra.

A growing number of chiropractors now utilize sophisticated noninvasive sensing devices such as the *surface electromyograph* or *EMG*. Electrodes are attached to various locations near the patient's spine and are then connected to the machine itself. The patient is instructed to perform a series of movements in a standing, sitting, and prone position that involve the use of the back muscles. By measuring electrical current in the spinal muscles, the EMG can indicate where spinal subluxations exist. Dr. Bertram Spector, former vice-president for research at the New York Chiropractic College, believes that surface electromyography enables the chiropractor to detect the location and extent of vertebral subluxations with a high degree of accuracy. Many practitioners agree.

Some chiropractors utilize heat and light in chiropractic analysis. *Thermography* is the more popular of the two. Through a process of scanning infrared heat emissions of the body, a color photograph can be produced that may indicate the presence of the vertebral subluxation complex.

Moiré contourography involves a unique process using the visible light spectrum and was first developed to provide three-dimensional information about soil-deformation and land-elevation contours. Through the analysis of distinct light patterns on various regions of the back, a skilled technician can determine the possible location and nature of a subluxation without having to use X-rays. Figure 7–3A shows how the "ideal" back appears through the moiré process. The symmetry of the concentric circles and bands at different elevations of the back indicates balance and harmony. Figure 7–3B, in contrast, shows a less-than-ideal back that reveals incomplete lines, circles, and bands. When analyzed by a specialist, the photograph would indicate a variety of structural disorders, including vertebral subluxation.

The X-Ray

Dr. Roberts then brought Ken into the X-ray room and took two pictures of his neck to determine the nature and extent of the suspected misalignment. After

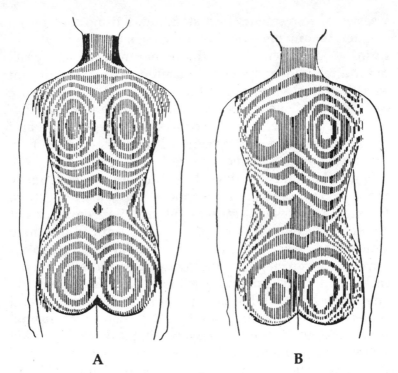

A   B

Figure 7–3. (A) An "ideal" back according to the moiré process, in-
dicating symmetry of concentric circles and bands. (B) A less-than-ideal
back revealing incomplete lines, circles, and bands. The areas of imbalance may indicate the presence of vertebral subluxations or other
spinal problems. From the Journal of Manipulative and Physiological Therapeutics. (Reprinted courtesy of Dr. Bertram Spector)

analyzing them, the earlier findings were confirmed: there
was a primary subluxation of the axis or second cervical
(2C) vertebra, which was putting pressure on a nerve. Dr.
Roberts said that this may have contributed to a stiff neck
as well as Ken's morning headaches, especially when Ken
slept on his right side. He also explained that other subluxations further down along the spine were the body's

attempts to compensate for this major misalignment and that they could be corrected as well.

A ten-week program of adjustments was drawn up that was typical of nonemergency, but chronic, cases such as Ken's: two adjustments a week for four weeks and one per week thereafter. (Other patients, such as recent accident victims, may begin with five adjustments a week; whereas patients with minor subluxations may start with one.) At the end of the tenth week, Ken's progress would be evaluated and he would probably need preventive maintenance only once a month thereafter. Chiropractors such as Dr. Roberts often recommend preventive care long after the original subluxations are corrected. Because chiropractic is based on the body's inborn ability to restore and maintain good health, regular chiropractic adjustments are seen as an important means of keeping the nervous system free of nerve interference and dis-ease.

Ken was pleased that Dr. Roberts's fee would be about half that of his medical doctor and would be covered by his health-insurance plan. After making appointments for future visits, Ken was ready to receive his first spinal adjustment.

The Adjustment

First Dr. Roberts took another temperature reading along the spinal column and wrote it in the record book. He then asked Ken to lie down on the table on his stomach, with his head turned to the right. At this point Ken tensed up a little, expecting a great deal of pain from the adjustment, but Dr. Roberts reassured him. Carefully applying light pressure on Ken's neck just below the right ear, he gave a sudden rapid downward thrust that made an audible "click" (see Figure 7–4). He did the same to a point on the upper back and had Ken, still in a prone

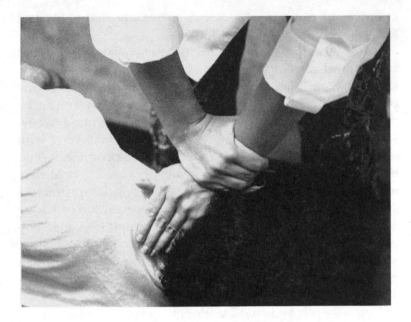

*Figure 7–4. A chiropractor adjusting the cervical area of the spine.
(Courtesy of the Palmer College of Chiropractic)*

position, cross his left leg over the other before he gave
the sacrum another rapid thrust. Although he felt a slight
tingling sensation in his head immediately after the adjustment, Ken was surprised to have felt no pain at all.
After a few minutes of rest, he got up from the table,
stretched, and observed that his neck felt better than it
had in years. Dr. Roberts replied that his response was far
from unusual. "Your cervical nerve was impinged for over
fifteen years," he said. "All we did was remove the interference."

Over the next ten weeks, Ken received a total of fourteen
chiropractic adjustments and began feeling better than he
had at any time since high school. He had more energy,
felt greater optimism about life, and had an exhilarating

absence of neck pain. He wondered why he had put up with it for so long.

This experience prompted Ken to ask how often a patient should be adjusted. There was no standard rule to follow, he was told. Schedules for adjustments have been known to vary from twice an hour (usually in an emergency situation when a high fever is present and the patient's life is in danger) to two or three times a week (for a patient with a chronic subluxation). After the initial problem is brought under control, preventive care is often scheduled once or twice a month.

Some chiropractors suggest that adjustments be discontinued as soon as symptoms disappear, but the majority believe that preventive maintenance should involve a long-term commitment. Many patients balk at the thought of receiving adjustments for years to come, but others feel that continuing maintenance (which has been likened to having periodic tune-ups and other regular maintenance performed on your car) will help preserve health and avoid the pain, disability, and financial costs involved when health care becomes disease care.

Dr. Roberts had given Ken a pamphlet by the second visit. It described an exercise program (similar to that in chapter 10) to help strengthen his spinal muscles and avoid subluxations. An extra-firm bed was recommended to replace Ken's old sagging mattress. The doctor also taught him the proper way to lift heavy, bulky objects in order to reduce the chances of subluxating his spine. Finally, Dr. Roberts encouraged Ken to improve his diet and suggested several books on nutrition and food preparation. He stressed that the better our diet, the less chance we have of subluxating the spine as a result of toxins found in heavily processed, devitalized foods.

Thanks to Dr. Roberts, Ken took a new interest in his health and joined a yoga class at the local community college. Through preventive care with Dr. Roberts and a personal program of exercise, diet, and stress management, Ken discovered that taking responsibility for his health was both easier and more pleasurable than he had imagined.

Although Ken may be a typical patient and Dr. Roberts a typical chiropractor who confines his practice largely to spinal adjustments alone, the profession itself is noted for variety and the ability to provide the kind of care patients want. Whereas some chiropractors rarely use X-rays and make judgments solely on their sense of touch and visual observation, others—who believe that X-rays show many spinal abnormalities that may require special caution— take a series of exposures before they adjust a patient and then follow-ups after every few months of care.

Although many chiropractors confine their practice largely to detecting spinal misalignments and correcting nerve interference, the majority of today's chiropractors may utilize blood tests, urinalysis, electrocardiograms, and other means to diagnose disease and pathology. After the diagnosis is completed, they often perform spinal adjustments along with a variety of adjunct therapies to treat the ailment or condition.

Hands-On Techniques

Chiropractors utilize a wide variety of adjustment techniques. Many are known by their initials—such as HIO, DNFT, and SOT—whereas others are named after their developers—such as Logan Basic, Gonstead, Pierce-Stilwagon, and Toftness. Although some are forceful and others involve a light touch, they are mostly done by hand and are designed primarily to remove nerve interference. Some chiropractors specialize in one technique (which was probably featured at their college); others use several methods depending on the nature and location of the subluxation. Most chiropractic techniques involve two concepts:

1. If a mechanical distortion is corrected, the body will restore normal nerve flow.
2. If nerve interference is removed, the body will restore its normal musculoskeletal structure.

Whatever the approach, chiropractic adjustments work. The following methods are among the most popular chiropractic techniques and are designed to bring about the precise and effective correction of spinal misalignments with a minimum of risk to the patient.

The Palmer Method. Developed by B. J. Palmer, this technique features a precise and rapid "toggle recoil" adjustment in which the chiropractor delivers a fast downward thrust to the subluxated vertebra followed by an immediate release of pressure. Palmer also introduced the famous hole-in-one adjustment, which focuses attention on the first cervical vertebra, or atlas (see Figure 7–5). He believed that once the misaligned atlas is adjusted, other subluxations—which may compensate for the atlas subluxation—will naturally realign themselves.

The Logan Basic Technique. In contrast to the Palmer, this technique stresses that "as goes the foundation of the building, so goes the structure." The developer of this early technique, Dr. Hugh B. Logan, maintained that misalignments at the base of the spine are the most important because the sacrum forms the foundation of the vertebral column. For this reason, chiropractors who use this popular method focus much of their attention on the sacrum.

The Sacro-Occipital Technique. Known in the profession as the SOT, this technique is viewed as a balance between the Palmer and Logan systems. Developed by Dr. M. B. de Jarnette, it involves both the sacrum and *occiput* (the back part of the skull) and is considered among the

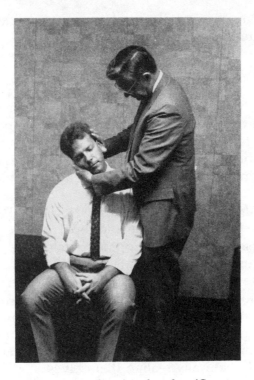

Figure 7–5. A chiropractor adjusting the atlas. (Courtesy of the Palmer College of Chiropractic)

most gentle of chiropractic techniques. Primarily designed to restore the flow of cerebrospinal fluid (so vital for nerve transmission and nutrition) at a point at the base of the skull, SOT is often utilized with an adjunct known as *cranial therapy*, described earlier.

Other Techniques. Both the Gonstead and Pierce-Stilwagon systems, for example, involve a specific "package" of different techniques involving the detection, analysis, and correction of vertebral subluxations. Some techniques, such as DNFT (Directional Non-Force Technique) and Toftness, involve a very light touch. In addition to utilizing a number of established forms of analysis, Network Chiropractic, developed by Donald Epstein, D.C., and described in *East West* magazine, allows for both dynamic and very light touch techniques. Adjustments are applied in a specific sequence according to the type and location of the subluxation, often with dramatic results.

Many chiropractors are familiar with a variety of chiropractic techniques and will choose what they feel will best help the individual patient. At a recent seminar I attended, one chiropractor joked that his favorite technique is "ATW: Anything That Works."

An Enviable Safety Record

Some degree of hazard exists in every technique, or every occupation for that matter, and something may go wrong despite every reasonable precaution whether we speak of chiropractic or any other health system. However, when we compare the percentage of mishaps between chiropractic and medical care, the chiropractor's safety record is an enviable one. Despite the AMA's attacks on the profession as useless, unscientific, and even dangerous, malpractice claims against chiropractors are extremely rare. The high rates of iatrogenic disease (illness as a consequence of drugs or surgery), inaccurate diagnosis, and unnecessary or botched surgical procedures and skyrocketing claims for medical malpractice show that the medical profession is hardly in a position to criticize other healthcare professions for lack of safety or effectiveness.

The respected New Zealand Commission referred to chiropractic as "remarkably safe." Despite its long vendetta against chiropractic, organized medicine in the United States has cited only a few documented cases of injury out of over 160 million chiropractic adjustments given each year.

Most of these were due to underlying pathologies such as tumors or artery conditions that the chiropractor was not able to recognize.

Isolated cases of accident and poor judgment have occurred. One case of malpractice years ago involved a chiropractor who promised to cure a little girl of cancer, convincing her parents not to send her to a medical doctor for treatment. After the child died, the chiropractor was convicted of second-degree murder. With rare exceptions such as this, practitioners will not claim to cure any disease, let alone a life-threatening illness such as cancer. They are trained to distinguish a chiropractic case from a medical one, and to refer the latter to the proper specialist for treatment.

Another area of concern involves the chiropractor's suggesting that patients discontinue taking medication. Unlike medical doctors, chiropractors do not have extensive training in pharmacology and drug therapy because they do not use medication in their practice. What they do know in these areas is often self-taught. For this reason there have been isolated cases of practitioners' recommending that patients discontinue certain medications, with unfortunate results. *Pennsylvania Medicine* cited one: "Under chiropractic care, an elderly woman with high blood pressure was advised to stop medication. Her blood pressure rose sharply and after a month she suffered a stroke."

Although such a case is rare, it illustrates that chiropractors are not in the position to recommend that patients discontinue medication. Very often, adjustments restore proper nerve transmission and the body's functions return to normal. However, responsible chiropractors leave such a decision to the patient and recommend that the medical doctor be consulted when such a step is contemplated. Since the resolution of the famous antitrust suit against the AMA (see chapter 3), it is likely that chiropractors and medical doctors will work together more closely than ever before. Joint practices, chiropractic residents in hospitals, and an increase in interprofessional consultation and referral are envisioned. The patient will be the ultimate beneficiary.

As mentioned earlier, adjustments performed by a licensed chiropractor provide maximum results with minimum risk. However, there is a danger with "chiropractic-type" manipulation performed by unqualified people. Although osteopaths, physical therapists, and some medical doctors receive instruction in the art of spinal manipulation, they have not received extensive training in chiropractic adjusting techniques, which only a chiropractor is qualified—and licensed—to perform. The New Zealand Commission addressed this issue, concluding that "chiropractors are the only health practitioners who are necessarily equipped by their education and training to carry out spinal manual therapy [chiropractic adjustments]." It added, "The responsibility for spinal manual therapy training, because of its specialized nature, should lie with the chiropractic profession."

PART THREE

*Beyond Spinal
Adjustments:
Constructive
Survival Values*

CHAPTER 8

Chiropractic Survival
Values

*E*arly in this century, B. J. Palmer developed
an important concept called *survival values* as an integral
part of the chiropractic philosophy. He taught that a survival value, in mathematical terms, is a *unit of adaptational
success* of the body to its environment, which permits the
state that we call health.

According to Dr. R. W. Stephenson's *Chiropractic Text
Book*, survival value is a unit of evolution. "Where there
is successful adaptation, there is no interruption to Innate's
[innate intelligence's] program." Palmer believed that chiropractic adjustments are a primary factor in promoting
what he called "constructive survival values" because they
enable the body to respond and adapt more easily to its
environment by restoring the integrity of the nervous
system.

Dr. Fred H. Barge, who has served as president of the
ICA and is a visiting professor at a number of chiropractic
colleges, stated: "It is time that [we] recognize the fact that
[the] body is in constant strife comprehending a hostile
environment. That imperative to the body's ability to function properly against external forces is the integrity of the
nervous system." He maintains that this will enable innate
intelligence to guide the individual to the highest level he
or she can reach as a human being.

Conversely, vertebral subluxations and other injuries
can lead to "destructive survival values." According to
Stephenson: "When there are subluxations or unusual adaptation, the law of destruction goes into effect, costing

the organization a loss of construction." Dr. Barge spoke of the effect of destructive survival values in his textbook *Life Without Fear*:

> The constructive survival values of the human system constantly strive to maintain a state of well being, and only when destructive forces become overbearing does the "momentum" of health break down and allow the body to exhibit the symptoms and signs of so-called sickness and disease.

According to Dr. Barge, *accumulated survival values* were originally used to describe the responses of the patient to chiropractic adjustments. Accumulated constructive survival values are weighed against the accumulated destructive survival values to help determine the likely prognosis to chiropractic care. This early concept is now an accepted part of holistic health philosophy. In *Who Gets Sick*, Blair Justice wrote:

> Risk factors—anything in our thinking, behavior, body, or environment that increases the likelihood of illness—are opposed by the "resistance resources" we possess. These may include an optimistic way of looking at life, a good social support system, and a strong set of genes. The balance between risk factors and resistance resources largely determines whether we get sick or stay healthy.

Diana, forty years of age, is suffering from rheumatoid arthritis. Her destructive survival values include the fact that she smokes a pack of cigarettes a day, has poor dietary habits, is thirty pounds overweight, and had a skiing accident ten years earlier that injured her spine. However, her constructive survival values include no spinal curvature, no degeneration of any spinal discs, a good sense of humor, and the will to get well. She is also a nondrinker. After evaluating her situation on a linear scale, her chiropractor saw a positive prognosis for her response to chiropractic care.

In contrast, George is a seventy-year-old retired contractor suffering from lung cancer. His destructive survival values include osteoporosis, diabetes, a serious neck injury during the war, the surgical removal of a gall bladder, and a history of alcohol abuse. His constructive survival values include an adequate income from a pension and investments, strong religious beliefs, a comfortable home in the country, and a loving wife. When observed from a linear, mechanistic viewpoint (which teaches that the body is the sum total of its parts), George's accumulated destructive values would outweigh the constructive values. As a result, his response to chiropractic care would normally be considered to be poor.

Yet when seen from a vitalistic viewpoint—which speaks of the tremendous healing potential of innate intelligence—George's situation is far from hopeless. According to Donald Epstein, D.C., "There is no sickness, disease, or symptom that cannot be the result of a reduced expression of your life force. The potential for destruction is released by the vertebral subluxation every single time." By removing nerve interference caused by the vertebral subluxation, George can gain access to his innate intelligence—which animates, motivates, heals, and coordinates his life. For this reason, vitalistic chiropractors never would presume to "second guess" innate intelligence regarding the ability of the patient to respond to chiropractic care, let alone recover from an illness. Their primary goal is not to evaluate or treat symptoms but to help the patient gain access to the body's innate wisdom and healing power.

Throughout much of this book we have seen that regular chiropractic care is important for good health because it insures the integrity of the nervous system. The nervous system, in turn, guides the function of every single organ, muscle, and tissue of our body. However, in addition to the positive effects that chiropractic can bring toward achieving constructive survival values in our lives, there are other aspects of health that can either enhance or limit the benefits of chiropractic care.

Some believe that as long as they receive regular adjustments they will remain healthy no matter how they abuse their bodies, such as the man who has smoked two packs of cigarettes a day for thirty years. Despite the fact that he may receive chiropractic adjustments every week, these may not be able to fully compensate for the harm done to his lungs, heart, and nervous system. The harmful chemical effects from cigarettes may increase the likelihood of subluxation as well.

Ideally, an entire book should be devoted to how we can achieve constructive survival values in our lives. Although not intended as a complete or comprehensive guide, this and the following two chapters will explore briefly some of the ways that we can take greater responsibility for our health by adopting a personal program for health maintenance as a complement to regular chiropractic care. The intent in presenting this material is to offer some ideas to promote constructive survival values rather than a program of hard-and-fast rules that everyone should follow. Like other health-care professionals, many chiropractors believe that healthy intentions and adaptation to stress, a wholesome and nutritious diet, and a program of safe and regular exercise will enhance the effectiveness of the care they provide. In addition, these factors help us achieve constructive survival values throughout our lives.

From Destructive to Constructive

First, let's compare some of the elements that influence these survival values. Though some may appear obvious, many of us don't pay attention to them in daily life. In one column, I offer a partial list of factors that lead to constructive survival values; in the other, a list of factors that can lead to destructive survival values. We often experience both positive and negative factors at the same time. Of course, the value of each factor varies according to each individual—for example, a big-city environment may be destructive for some people whereas others thrive in it. Through the daily gain of constructive or destructive survival values we help determine not only our health and overall life expectancy but also our ability to function at a high level of energy, creativity, and personal satisfaction.

Constructive	Destructive
ability to relax	anxiety, tension
chiropractic adjustments	vertebral subluxations
eating "just enough"	undereating, overeating
pure, nutritious foods	refined, adulterated foods
regular exercise	physical inactivity
pure air	air pollution
optimistic view of life	negativity, depression
good posture habits	poor posture habits
good relationships	poor relationships/isolation
satisfaction at work	frustration at work
sense of humor	overly serious
correct weight	more than ten pounds overweight or underweight

In the following case history, we will examine constructive life-style factors and destructive factors. See how the two balance out in the life of Suzanne, a chiropractic patient from California.

Suzanne is an executive who enjoys her work at a public relations firm in downtown Los Angeles. After a good night's rest, she goes jogging with her husband and devotes fifteen minutes to meditation and relaxation. She eats a good breakfast of whole-grain cereal, fresh fruit, and yogurt, kisses and hugs her husband Tom good-bye, and drives to work on a crowded, slow-moving freeway.

On entering the office, she learns that her company is about to lose an important account, and she is asked to convince her client to stay. After a flurry of tense conferences with her angry boss and several frustrating phone calls to arrange a meeting with her client, the two women finally agree to meet that evening for dinner. Suzanne manages to take a fifteen-minute break to do some stretching exercises while her secretary makes the restaurant reservations.

Leaving work early, Suzanne decides to walk along a quiet route through the park to her chiropractor's office for her biweekly adjustment. Although feeling some anxiety about the dinner meeting, Suzanne believes she can persuade the client not to leave.

She meets the client in a quiet restaurant with relaxed surroundings. Suzanne orders a light meal with one glass of wine. Despite lingering fears of losing the account, her sense of humor puts both Suzanne and her client at ease. The meeting goes well, and although no final decision has been reached the client agrees to seriously review her company's wish to seek another agency.

Exhausted, Suzanne returns home late at night but is greeted with a warm hug and kiss by her husband. After Suzanne and Tom share the day's events, they give each other a relaxing massage before going to bed.

Suzanne's day was not without what most of us would perceive as negative factors: the morning traffic, inner-city pollution, a crisis at work, and anxiety about keeping the client. However, because she also had positive things working for her that day (such as a good diet, physical affection from her husband, regular exercise, relaxation, a sense of humor, and a chiropractic adjustment) she was more able to transform negative challenges into opportunities leading to constructive survival values. Although each factor cannot be precisely weighed on a mathematical scale, Suzanne would appear to have finished her day with a net gain in survival value, which had a constructive effect on her well-being. The positive momentum that is built from day to day helps her to deal better with the often difficult challenges of everyday living.

At the same time, we need to remember that words such as *constructive* and *destructive*, or *positive* and *negative*, are highly subjective and depend on each individual's case. In addition, what we perceive as negative in the short-term can lead to constructive survival values in the long-term. Let me use a personal example.

Eighteen months before beginning work on this book, I experienced a period of intense stress. This "stress package" involved the death of my mother, troubles with other family members, unexpected expenses, difficulties as executor of the estate, and a fast-approaching deadline to complete a book for an anxious publisher. Like many other men raised in this country, I repressed my grief, anger, and frustration under a facade of strength, detachment, and efficiency.

While moving some furniture several months later, I suffered an abdominal hernia. My symptoms included pain and fatigue, especially when standing for more than ten minutes at a time, and they led to decreased mobility, overeating, and weight gain. I felt that I was falling apart physically, and I experienced anger, frustration, and even a feeling of martyrdom at my situation. These problems and negative attitudes would be considered by most people (including myself) as destructive survival values. After more than a year of discomfort and limitation, I finally had the hernia surgically repaired.

Looking back, I believe that this apparently negative situation brought many benefits. During a period of intense stress, I became more aware of my body and its need to be nurtured and treated with respect. The decreased mobility forced me to relax. Spending more time at home, I created a more pleasant working and living environment. In addition, I felt freer to ask friends for help and received needed sympathy and concern for my condition. As a result, I have learned how to better look after myself.

Finally, I believe that much of the repressed grief, anger, and frustration surrounding my mother's death and my dealing with her estate was "channeled" through the hernia. In retrospect, these feelings should ideally have been expressed without physical symptoms. At the same time, a greater degree of repression might have affected my heart or other major organ with more dramatic results. Of course, I would not recommend that everyone experience a hernia when having difficulty dealing with personal problems, but I believe that mine helped keep me relatively healthy when I was unable to deal with what I perceived as an overwhelming situation. I now appreciate that symptoms need not be seen solely in a negative light, because they can open the door to new insights and opportunities for growth.

A genuine desire to be well is a major ingredient in attaining constructive survival values, as B. J. Palmer taught years ago. This reflects inner attitudes that promote and enhance health in obedience to our inner intuitive faculties, which tell us (often very subtly) that our body's wisdom needs to function without psychological or emotional interference. According to O. Carl Simonton, M.D., Stephanie Matthews-Simonton, and James Creighton in their important book for cancer patients, *Getting Well Again*: "The unconscious mind contains priceless resources that can be mobilized for personal growth and healing. Indeed, throughout the history of psychological study, theoreticians have proposed the existence of a 'center' in the psyche which directs, regulates, and influences the course of the individual's life."

Chiropractic care can help us become more responsive

to this inner wisdom, and chiropractors recommend that we make an effort to be open to our intuitive feelings about physical and psychological needs and then use common sense to do what is necessary to fulfill them.

Table 8–1 is a "habits list" and is one way to see how you look at health. It can help you pinpoint your positive

Table 8–1. A Habits List

Habit	Once a month or less	Few times a month	Few times a week or daily
1. Engage in sports, jogging, calisthenics, dancing, etc.			
2. Walk ½ mile or more			
3. Go out socially			
4. Meditate or pray			
5. Have a period of quiet, unthinking relaxation			
6. Have enough sleep			
7. Feel joyous or at peace			
8. Engage in pleasurable sexual activity			
9. Give/receive physical affection			
10. Feel anxious, fearful, or under pressure			
11. Eat too much			
12. Smoke cigarettes			
13. Feel depressed			
14. Feel physical pain			
15. Be exhausted from work			
16. Take mind-altering drugs			
17. Feel resentful			
18. Drink enough alcohol to get high			
19. Drink 2 or more cups of coffee a day			

feelings and also those areas that need attention. Complete the table, and after you are done ask why you responded as you did. Do your answers reflect a positive statement toward life? Do they say no to life? What are the underlying reasons behind the yes or the no?

The first nine categories—if experienced daily or several times a week—generally reveal feelings of positive intent toward health. The latter ten tend to reflect unresolved issues and a possible negative intent toward health. When you discover a negative habit or situation, ask if it is a "pseudosolution" to fulfill certain real needs. For example, does overeating serve as a pseudosolution for other forms of pleasure, such as sharing physical affection with another? Does it help to avoid feelings of sadness or anxiety? After finding the truth, seek out positive alternatives to satisfy these needs that will not be stressful to your health.

Managing Stress

Stress is a normal part of life according to Hans Selye, author of *Stress Without Distress*. It is not just nervous tension but rather the body's response to any demand made on it. A family argument *or* a pleasurable experience such as watching a sunset can produce stress. Although we would be dead without any stress, Selye points out that our ability to adapt to stress determines our level of health. Poor adaptation leads to *distress*, which has been linked to a wide range of health problems such as hypertension, migraine headaches, heart disease, ulcers, and even cancer.

Chiropractors believe that an unobstructed nervous system, free from vertebral subluxations, enables us to deal better with the tensions of our inner and outer environment, whereas subluxations make adaptation more difficult. According to Dr. Donald Epstein in the *Digest of*

Chiropractic Economics, "If vertebral subluxations are not present, spinal tension will reduce, allowing the individual to recover from stress. In a subluxated state, the spinal tone may persist and actually intensify, remaining long after the stress has left, due to a nonadaptive nervous system."

At the same time, chiropractors also are aware that poor emotional adaptation to stress can produce vertebral subluxations. In a vicious circle, the nerve interference caused by these subluxations can, over time, further inhibit the body's ability to adapt to stress. Although regular chiropractic adjustments can correct vertebral subluxations, we can prevent their frequent occurrence by dealing with stress in positive ways.

Professionals from various health fields have suggested a number of ways to deal with stress: going for a walk or run, enjoying music, participating in a sport or hobby, reading a book, or working in a garden. Other approaches may be less conventional, but equally effective. Norman Cousins, in his book *Anatomy of an Illness,* told how ten minutes of belly laughter at frequent intervals (he saw Marx Brothers movies and old "Candid Camera" television shows) helped him overcome a life-threatening disease. Humor shouldn't be used as a total escape from life, but integrating "laugh therapy" into each day can relieve tension. B. J. Palmer recognized its value. He had the following message painted over the men's urinal in one of the washrooms at the Palmer School of Chiropractic: LESSON NUMBER NINE: DON'T TAKE YOURSELF TOO DAMN SERIOUSLY.

Another enjoyable way to deal with daily tension is "hug therapy." Dr. David Bresler of the UCLA Pain Control Unit in Los Angeles prescribes a minimum of four hugs a day for men and women to relieve everyday nervous tension.

A simple, effective exercise that releases stress involves a selective tensing up and relaxing of voluntary muscles of the body. Though not measured by scientific instruments until recently, the benefits of this exercise include a decrease in muscle tension (which can reduce the possibility of vertebral subluxation), heartbeat, oxygen consumption, blood pressure, and respiratory rate. Other methods were introduced by Dr. Herbert Benson in his best-seller *The Relaxation Response* and by Dr. Simonton in his *Getting Well Again*. (Details of these and other books about stress management and relaxation can be found in the References section.)

Breathing

Indian yogis have known the secret of deep rhythmic breathing for thousands of years. In addition to its ability to reduce muscle tension, it is now recognized by medical doctors as an effective way to improve blood circulation, decrease heartbeat, and lower blood pressure. Considered to be a complete relaxation technique in itself, deep breathing also can serve as a foundation for several aspects of meditation, such as creative visualization, concentration, prayer, receptivity, and sending good feelings to others.

Communing with Innate Intelligence

Meditation not only helps us to adapt better to stress but it can also help us get in touch with our inner wisdom. According to early teachings, the meaning of meditation is "to bring to the center." In chiropractic terms, this means the core where our innate intelligence resides. Some chiropractors believe that meditation can help prevent subluxations caused by nervous tension and can increase the time we can "hold" a chiropractic adjustment.

There are many other practices that lead to constructive survival values. Choosing an enjoyable career or avocation, learning to enjoy work, taking up a hobby, learning how to express feelings, learning how to confront others in a spirit of love without holding a grudge, and learning how to create pleasure in daily life (taking time for a walk, visiting good friends, treating yourself to a bubble bath, or giving yourself the vacation or special gift you've always wanted). Although these methods and enjoyments may appear frivolous at first glance, they reflect a deeper, positive intent to avoid tension, disharmony, and fatigue. They create constructive survival values in our lives.

Healthy intentions are an integral part of the chiropractic process because they lead us to seek preventive—as opposed to crisis—care. By consciously working to achieve constructive survival values in daily life, we help our chiropractor keep us free from vertebral subluxations: a primary cause of dis-ease. We actively participate in our wellbeing by recognizing and transforming destructive beliefs and unhealthy practices, which create subluxations and inhibit our natural healing process, into attitudes and practices that help us enjoy life to the fullest.

CHAPTER 9

Eating for Life and Spinal Health

Diet and nutrition have been of increasing concern among health-care professionals, but chiropractic's focus is unique. Like mainstream dietitians and clinical nutritionists, chiropractors believe that good nutrition is essential to health and overall well-being. At the same time, they are concerned about the impact of nutrition on the development and maintenance of nerves, muscles, and bones. According to the *Official ICA Policy Statement on Chiropractic* passed in 1982: "The Chiropractic clinical application also includes . . . nutritional advice for the maintenance of health, especially as it relates to the soundness of the neuromuscular skeletal structures." Some practitioners believe as well that poor dietary habits and toxins from alcohol, food additives, and pesticide residues in food are factors that can lead to subluxations of the spine. Degenerative diseases such as diabetes, atherosclerosis, and arthritis may follow later in life as a result.

For these reasons, good nutrition always has been an important concern of chiropractic. In the early 1900s, several of the training colleges taught nutrition and dietetics as part of their regular curriculum, whereas most other colleges—and medical schools in particular—believed that nutrition was of minor importance. This attitude among medical schools has slowly begun to change, but the chiropractor's training in clinical nutrition far surpasses that of the average medical student today. Some chiropractic colleges offer postgraduate diplomas in clinical nutrition, and the American Chiropractic Association maintains a

Council of Nutrition to keep members abreast of the latest developments in the field.

One of the first chiropractic books to discuss diet and nutrition was the previously cited *Chiropractic Text Book* by R. W. Stephenson, a professor at the Palmer School (now College) of Chiropractic. Although concern about artificial food additives and environmental pollution did not capture the public interest until recently, Dr. Stephenson addressed these issues seventy years ago: "Anything made or prepared artificially and then introduced into the body, against which Innate rebels, is a poison. Foods, air, or water when they have been 'doctored' are poisons."

B. J. Palmer also took a strong interest in nutrition but warned that prescribing specific diets was contrary to the basic philosophy of chiropractic. He believed that each person had unique dietary needs and could intuitively choose the needed foods if given the chance (provided that nerve supply was unobstructed by subluxations). He claimed that the educated intelligence of the chiropractor could not presume to know what kind of diet the patient's innate intelligence required for the body's optimum health.

Although Palmer's point is well taken, few chiropractors believe that innate intelligence should be the only guide to proper nutrition. As Stephenson wrote, "The nourishment of the body should be governed by Innate Intelligence, with the cooperation of the educated mind. The educated mind should serve as a cooperative function and not as a hindrance to innate mind, in the selection of food for the body."

However, Stephenson also was quoted as having said: "A sick person's abnormal educated mind will not allow him to use common sense; therefore somebody else's common sense must be used." Many practitioners believe that as primary health-care providers they should be concerned with the whole of the patient's health and should not confine themselves to only one area of health. They maintain that since nutritional guidance is not offered by most health practitioners, chiropractors have a responsibility to offer the commonsense advice that is the result of their professional training. Therefore, they fill a vital need that is often ignored.

There are at least forty different nutrients—including protein, carbohydrates, fats, vitamins, and minerals— needed in the human diet. Many chiropractors believe that a diet rich in essential nutrients will not only nourish the body as a whole but also supply essential elements for the maintenance of nerves, bones, and muscles, including those involving the spine. Some teach that the role of nutrition and the vertebral subluxation is a two-way affair: on one hand, a vertebral subluxation and the resulting nerve interference can affect digestion and the absorption of nutrients; on the other, poor dietary habits and especially the ingestion of toxins can be factors that increase the possibility for a vertebral subluxation to occur. As a result, people with healthy nerve tissue, well-nourished muscles, and bones rich in calcium and other essential minerals may be less likely to be subject to subluxations of the spine. On the following pages, we will explore some of the ways that nutrition can affect the nervous system, muscles, and bones.

Nutrients and the Central Nervous System

Because of its high metabolic rate and its importance in controlling and maintaining body functions, the central nervous system is profoundly influenced by diet and nutrition. For example, fat provides essential fatty acids for the normal development of nerves, and various amino acids (the building blocks of protein) as well as minerals aid in normal nerve transmission. Deficiencies have been linked to poor neural function.

Certain B vitamins are important for healthy nerves. Thiamin is essential for proper nerve function, and deficiencies can lead to illness in both the brain and peripheral nervous system. Vitamin B_{12} is essential for maintaining healthy nerve tissue, and deficiencies can affect spinal cord tracts, the optic nerve, and fatty acid metabolism of the peripheral nervous system.

According to C. E. Sawyer, Ph.D., of the Northwestern College of Chiropractic, neurological function is influenced by changes in neurotransmitter synthesis induced by diet. Certain amino acids and iron are among the nutrients essential to this process. Children with iron deficiency have revealed a short attention span, behavioral problems, and other developmental problems related to a poorly functioning nervous system.

Finally, certain elements have been found to have an effect on the nervous systems of some individuals. Lead and food additives containing vasoactive amines (such as monosodium glutamate, or MSG) have been linked with hyperactivity in children through their action on the central nervous system.

Nutrients and Strong Bones

Good nutrition is needed to maintain healthy bones. Calcium makes up some 99 percent of our skeletal structure, and phosphorus is essential for bone strength. Rickets and osteomalacia are primary results of deficiencies of these minerals, both resulting in soft bones. Osteoporosis—the overall loss of bone mass—is also due to a deficiency of calcium. Magnesium is a catalyst to help the body utilize calcium. In addition to calcium, minerals that are found in the discs between the vertebrae include sodium, potassium, magnesium, and iron. Their absorption is affected by the free movement of joints.

Vitamins too are important for healthy bones. Vitamin C, for example, is responsible for the health and maintenance of collagen, a gelatinlike protein found in teeth, bones, and connective tissue. Vitamin C stabilizes the structure of collagen and is essential for the healing of wounds and fractures. Vitamin D promotes the normal calcification of bones.

In his paper on nutrition and the musculoskeletal system presented at the 1986 Symposium on Nutrition and Chiropractic, Dr. Louis J. Freedman of Palmer College stated: "An adequate supply of water, carbohydrates, protein, fat, essential vitamins, and trace minerals is important for normal growth in the child and for maintenance and repair in the adult."

Muscles and Good Nutrition

Skeletal muscles make up about 40 percent of our body mass and are responsible for the movement of the skeletal system. Strong, healthy muscles are of special concern to chiropractors, since they provide support and protect the spine. Literally hundreds of muscles are attached to each vertebra, and permit free movement of the entire body.

Protein is essential for proper muscle structure, and deficiencies can lead to muscle deterioration. Carbohydrates and fats are also important sources of energy used by the skeletal muscles, and certain vitamins, especially vitamin E, are specifically linked to muscle maintenance and repair.

Eating for Health

The first step a chiropractor may take in creating a dietary program is to determine the patient's health history. Special attention is given to any nutrition-related disorders, such as constipation, diabetes, or high blood pressure, as well as to such problems as being overweight or underweight and having skin disorders or insomnia. You might be asked about life-style and physical activity: "Do you sit at a desk all day long?" "Do you exercise daily?" "How far do you walk to the supermarket?" "Do you perform housework or other physical tasks?"

The chiropractor may suggest that the patient prepare a nutritional diary in order to find the amount and variety of foods he or she consumes during the week. There is no standard form for such a diary, but Eleanor Gilpatrick, Ph.D., tells students taking her "Ecology for Health" course at Hunter College in New York City to set up a weekly chart. Her instructions are in Table 9-1.

To provide more effective nutritional guidance, some chiropractors, either directly or through collaboration with a certified dietitian, want to learn about their patients' deeper attitudes regarding certain foods. You may be asked to fill out a questionnaire on which you list the foods you consume, how often you consume them, how you feel about your food intake, and which foods you try to include or avoid in your daily diet. An example of such a survey is shown in Table 9-2.

Good nutrition is our personal responsibility, and practitioners feel they need to be aware of their patients' underlying intent toward food and health before a particular nutritional program that will work can be recommended. A primary concern among many chiropractors is the adulterated and unhealthy foods that make up the basic diet of the majority of people living in industrialized countries such as ours. Some feel that such food can produce vertebral subluxations, in addition to helping us put on weight, stimulating us when we are tired, and making us numb when we are tense. They warn that when we lose touch with our body's innate intelligence, we are unable to give it what it really needs.

Many people select "empty calorie" foods such as pastry

Table 9–1. Nutritional Diary

Fill in the food you eat each day. Try to list what you eat as soon as you eat it. This includes breakfast, lunch, dinner, between-meal snacks, coffee breaks, bedtime snacks, etc. Include coffee, tea, water, alcoholic beverages, candy, and "munchies" in front of the TV set. List everything, even what you may not be too happy about.

Day	Breakfast	Between Meals	Lunch	Between Meals	Dinner	Between Meals
Wed.						
Thur.						
Fri.						
Sat.						
Sun.						
Mon.						
Tues.						

Reprinted courtesy of Dr. Eleanor Gilpatrick

made with refined flour and sugar, sugary drinks, and candy, which are high in calories but low in essential vitamins and minerals. Consumption of these in place of foods such as whole grains, fresh fruits and vegetables, legumes, seeds, and nuts is of concern to nutritionists who observe that many of us become fat and undernourished at the same time.

Nearly 15 percent of the population is considered to weigh 30 percent or more over their desirable weight by the United States government. This is of concern among chiropractors. Normally, the spine is held in place by ligaments and muscles that efficiently support it. Being overweight (especially with what is known as a "potbelly") disturbs the spine's proper muscle tone because the abdomen needs more support. As a result, subluxations occur. Any "extra baggage" subjects the entire body to unnecessary stress and strain that can limit our ability to enjoy a long, healthy life.

For these reasons, the American Chiropractic Association Council on Nutrition prepared the "Ten Most Unwanted List." These foods and other items are consumed in large quantities by the majority of Americans and should be replaced by substances that are healthier:

1. White refined sugar and candy
2. Alcoholic beverages
3. Coffee
4. Cola beverages and artificially colored drinks
5. Artificially flavored products with too many preservatives added
6. "Junk" foods and snacks
7. White-flour products
8. Hot dogs and some fast-food items
9. Tobacco
10. Prepared foods, such as TV dinners and numerous other "quick" convenience foods (that are high in sodium, fat, and artificial flavorings or colorings)

Table 9–2. Health Survey

INTAKE

Check the items that best describe your *current* intake and attitudes.

		Frequency			Attitude	
	Never or Rarely	Few Times per Month	Several Times per Week or Daily	Try to Avoid	Try to Include
1. Meat	—	—	—	—	—
2. Fish, fowl	—	—	—	—	—
3. Eggs	—	—	—	—	—
4. Milk, cheese, yogurt	—	—	—	—	—
5. Whole grains	—	—	—	—	—
6. Peas, beans, lentils	—	—	—	—	—
7. Nuts, seeds	—	—	—	—	—
8. Fresh or dried fruit	—	—	—	—	—
9. Cooked fruits, vegetables	—	—	—	—	—
10. Raw vegetables	—	—	—	—	—
11. Bran, roughage	—	—	—	—	—
12. Vitamin supplements	—	—	—	—	—
13. Mineral supplements	—	—	—	—	—
14. Protein supplements	—	—	—	—	—
15. Water	—	—	—	—	—
16. Sugar as additive, any form	—	—	—	—	—
17. Coffee, caffeine, tea, other caffeine drinks	—	—	—	—	—
18. Alcohol	—	—	—	—	—
19. Aspirin and other nonprescription medicine(s)	—	—	—	—	—
20. Refined grains, starches	—	—	—	—	—

		Frequency		Attitude	
	Never or Rarely	*Few Times per Month*	*Several Times per Week or Daily*	*Try to Avoid*	*Try to Include*
21. Other processed foods	—	—	—	—	—
22. Salt as additive	—	—	—	—	—
23. Food coloring	—	—	—	—	—
24. Food preservatives	—	—	—	—	—
25. Saturated, hydrogenated fats, oils	—	—	—	—	—
26. Polyunsaturated fats	—	—	—	—	—
27. Prescription medicine(s): (Fill in which)	—	—	—	—	—
	—	—	—	—	—
28. Mind-altering drugs: (Fill in which)	—	—	—	—	—
	—	—	—	—	—

29. Do you currently smoke? Check one below:
Never _____ Rarely _____ About half pack per day _____
About pack per day _____ More than pack per day _____

FEELINGS ABOUT INTAKE:

	Good and Healthful	*Fairly Healthful*	*Not Good, and Would Like Help*	*Not Good, and Don't Want Help*
1. My food intake is:	—	—	—	—
2. My liquid intake is:	—	—	—	—
3. My food supplement intake is:	—	—	—	—
4. My alcohol intake is:	—	—	—	—
5. My use of medications is:	—	—	—	—
6. My use of drugs is:	—	—	—	—
7. My use of tobacco is:	—	—	—	—
8. My overall diet is:	—	—	—	—
9. Conditions under which I eat, when I eat, and the time I give to eating are:	—	—	—	—

A Chiropractic Diet?

It is difficult to find two chiropractors who completely agree on what an optimum diet should be. Some think that nutrition is simply not their concern, and refer patients to a professional nutritionist. Among those providing nutritional advice, there is a tendency to avoid extremes, with the chiropractor working with each individual patient to formulate a balance compatible with his or her needs. Such diets are generally low in fat, refined sugar, salt, and heavily processed foods. They may contain fewer animal products than we are accustomed to, yet they provide sufficient vitamins, minerals, proteins, dietary fiber, and other food elements essential for good health.

Chiropractors who participated in the 1986 Symposium on Nutrition and Chiropractic at Palmer College suggested that we adopt the following recommendations offered in *Dietary Guidelines for Americans*, published by the U.S. Department of Agriculture and the U.S. Department of Health and Human Services the previous year:

1. Eat a variety of foods.
2. Maintain desirable weight.
3. Avoid too much fat, saturated fat, and cholesterol.
4. Eat foods with adequate starch and fiber.
5. Avoid too much sugar.
6. Avoid too much sodium.
7. If you drink alcoholic beverages, do so in moderation.

These guidelines are considered very conservative, and tend to leave much to interpretation. For clarity, we will examine these recommendations in more detail, based on the suggestions given at the 1986 symposium mentioned above.

Eat a variety of foods. It was recommended that we should include fruits, vegetables, whole grain cereals, enriched breads, and a source of dairy products (such as milk, cheese, or yogurt) daily. Fish, lean meats, poultry, eggs, and dried beans or peas were included as good sources of protein.

Maintain desirable weight. By eating food slowly and chewing it carefully, taking smaller portions and avoiding second helpings, and eating fewer fatty foods and less sugar, sweets, and alcoholic beverages, we can maintain control over the number of calories we consume. In place of these undesirable foods, we should consume fruits, vegetables, and whole grains. Finally, by increasing physical activity, we burn up more calories.

Avoid too much fat, saturated fat, and cholesterol. Fried foods, fatty meats, butter, cream, lard, margarine, and palm and coconut oils are all high in fat and cholesterol and their consumption should be reduced. Eggs and organ meats (such as liver) should be eaten sparingly, if at all. Lean meat, fish, poultry, and legumes (such as dried beans, peas, and lentils) tend to be lower in fat and are recommended protein sources. Boil, bake, or broil your food rather than fry it.

Eat foods with adequate starch and fiber. Good sources of fiber and starch include whole grain breads and cereals (including oat bran), whole grain pasta, fresh fruits and vegetables, and dried peas, beans, and lentils.

Avoid too much sugar. In addition to reducing obvious sources of sugar such as table sugar (white or brown), molasses, and honey, there are hidden sources of sugar that find their way into a myriad of consumer products— cookies, crackers, cakes, beverages (including fruit punch, juice, and soft drinks), canned fruits, vegetables and soup, and breakfast cereals. If the ingredients listed on the label begin with sugar, fructose, dextrose, glucose, or corn syrup, too much of the product is made up of sugar. Read the labels.

Avoid too much sodium. Like sugar, sodium is consumed in excess by most Americans. In addition to the table salt we add to food ourselves, many products, including potato chips, frozen dinners, pickled foods, soy sauce, processed cheese spreads, salted nuts, and canned soups and vegetables, often contain added salt. Read the labels. In addition to limiting the amount of salt we add to foods, herbs and spices (some of which are commercially prepared) are recommended substitutes.

If you drink alcoholic beverages, do so in moderation. Alcoholic beverages are generally high in calories and low in nutrients. People who consume large quantities of alcohol run the risks of addiction, becoming overweight, and developing vitamin and mineral deficiencies. Alcohol has been linked also to birth defects when consumed by pregnant women. Nutritionists tend to agree that one or two drinks per day do no harm to average adults (providing that they are not pregnant). Twelve ounces of beer, five ounces of wine, and an ounce and a half of whisky, rum, or vodka count as one drink.

Aside from elaborating on these general recommendations, the participants of the Symposium on Nutrition and Chiropractic did not make any specific suggestions or diet plans. However, William Harris, Ph.D., of the Cleveland Chiropractic College in Kansas City, commented briefly on the government guidelines:

The dietary guidelines can be summed up by saying the closer a person comes to a vegetarian diet, the more healthful that diet is. A diet that is composed of foods that grow from the ground is low in fat, low in calories, low in cholesterol, high in fiber, high in vitamins and minerals and high in complex carbohydrates. All these components put together spell healthy eating for the typical American. Every chiropractic doctor should be aware of these guidelines.*

In an era when much of our food is transported over large distances, stored for long periods of time, and grown in soil that is often deficient in minerals, many nutritionists feel that even the most balanced diet does not provide adequate nutrition. For this reason, they suggest the use of commercial vitamin and mineral supplements. The American Chiropractic Association has advocated their use as they pertain to chiropractic: "Vitamin and mineral supplementation can, if professionally supervised, serve to prevent the onset or assuage the existence of some types of dysfunction of the nervous system and other tissues." With this in mind, a growing number of practitioners advise the use of—and often sell—preparations of commercial vitamin and mineral supplements to chiropractic patients.

One final note: The nutritional expertise of chiropractors varies greatly. The bulk of their training may be limited to what they learned in chiropractic college, although this represents more than a medical doctor receives. Some may have taken an extra course or two on nutrition, which does not necessarily qualify a chiropractor as a nutritionist. A certain number of practitioners have earned postgraduate degrees in nutrition, either in chiropractic colleges or other accredited institutions. Those who have a proven expertise in nutrition can use the title "Diplomate of the American Chiropractic Board of Nutrition." If your chiropractor is qualified to provide nutritional counseling, he or she can suggest a dietary program for your particular needs. Many

*The entire Proceedings of the Symposium on Nutrition and Chiropractic, 1986 is available from the Palmer College of Chiropractic, 1000 Brady St., Davenport, IA 52803.

chiropractors refer their patients to certified nutritionists for in-depth nutritional counseling and advice.

Know your chiropractor's qualifications before you rely on him or her for nutritional guidance and avoid the hit-and-miss approach to nutrition that many so-called experts practice today. If you have a special problem that goes beyond the expertise of a chiropractor, he or she has an obligation to refer you to the appropriate specialist. Nutrition is a major part of our taking responsibility for our health. Your local bookseller or librarian can recommend books on diet and nutrition, as well as exciting and interesting cookbooks with recipes from around the world.

Chapter 10

Staying in Shape: Exercise for a Healthy Spine

Chiropractic teaches that overall health is, in part, a measure of the well-being of the spinal column. In addition to correcting misalignments, many chiropractors recommend regular exercise to strengthen spinal muscles and thus help reduce vertebral subluxations. Like healthy intentions and a nutritious diet, a regular program of exercise, posture development, and proper lifting can promote constructive survival values in our lives and keep us on the road to good health.

Exercise: Points to Consider

Every form of exercise provides some benefits, but not all offer the same advantages. Jogging, skiing, rugby, wrestling, dance, and the martial arts are excellent body conditioners, but from a chiropractic point of view may be too strenuous on joints, ligaments, and the spinal column.

Jogging, for example, reduces tension, improves our ability to deliver oxygen to all parts of the body, increases muscle tone, and improves blood circulation. However, it jars the body, particularly the spine, and can be a cause of vertebral subluxation. Sports such as snow skiing, football, and wrestling often lead to strains in the spinal muscles and bruising injuries to the spinal column itself.

Chiropractors generally do not discourage their patients from practicing these forms of exercise, but advise that sports equipment should be in good order, overexertion should be avoided, and complete spinal examinations should be received before beginning a sport to determine if there are any physical limitations that could make such exercise dangerous. They also recommend an immediate visit after experiencing any mishaps.

Stretch for Spinal Health

Stretching exercises are among the finest body conditioners and are favored by chiropractors for themselves and their patients. When performed with knowledge and care, they are excellent for firming and toning the muscles of the arms, legs, shoulders, neck, and back. They also firm up abdominal muscles that are directly involved in preventing spinal disorders. According to Thomas Pipes and Paul Vodak, authors of *The Pipes Fitness Test and Prescription:* "When your abdominal strength and endurance are poor, the lower intestines, which are contained in a supporting membrane that attaches to the lower spine, protrude outward, causing disruptive stress on the spine. With continued stress, the backbone eventually distorts, pinching various nerves."

The most popular stretching exercises are featured in the ancient practice of hatha-yoga. Chiropractors often recommend yoga because it helps us relax, improves muscle tone, strengthens the abdominal and spinal muscles, and enables the spine to be more flexible and respond better to everyday stress and strain. There are a number of fine courses on hatha-yoga available in book and record stores. Classes in yoga and other stretching exercises are offered in most communities. If taught by a qualified instructor, the benefits can be great. A chiropractor offered the following advice: "Don't overdo it, and don't force the exercises by straining the muscles or by making sudden movements. Your body is made to move gracefully, and you don't have to force it into positions that cause pain and discomfort."

Nine Daily Exercises for Spinal Health

Many chiropractors tailor an exercise program to the individual needs of the patient, often drawing the best features from different exercise systems. The following ones were created by a chiropractor and are especially designed to strengthen the muscles of the neck, abdomen, and back. They reduce tension while improving muscle tone and strength, and are intended to minimize the onset of vertebral subluxations and to improve the effectiveness of chiropractic adjustments. Perform these as often as you like, although twice a day is considered ideal. Each can be done by itself or in a group, but all nine should be performed in order to obtain maximum benefits.

Before starting any exercise program, speak to your chiropractor about any possible physical limitations you may have. Those offered here should not cause any pain and can be performed by people of all ages. However, if one or more of the exercises cause discomfort, it may indicate a spinal problem.

Neck Exercises

1. Cervical (neck) Extension. In a standing position, slowly nod your head backward until you feel a firm pressure at the base of the head (as opposed to letting your head drop as far as it will go). Hold this position for a slow count of three. Slowly bring your head to an erect position once more. Repeat five times. Increase the number daily until you can do twenty. Like the following exercise, the cervical extension helps strengthen neck muscles and improve their general tone. (See Figure 10–1.)

2. *Cervical Flexion.* In a standing position, gently nod your head forward onto your chest and hold to the count of three. Make sure to avoid any strain of the neck muscles. Hold this position for another count of three. Slowly bring your head erect. Repeat five times. Slowly increase the number daily until you can do twenty. (See Figure 10–2.)

3. *Cervical Left and Right.* In a standing position, turn your head slowly to the left without straining or rolling your head up and down. Hold this position for 3 seconds. Bring your head back to the center, and rest. Then slowly turn your head to the right, hold, and bring your head back to center once more. Repeat five times. Gradually increase the repetitions daily until twenty are achieved. The goal of this exercise is to increase the lateral range of motion of the neck and improve muscle tone. (See Figure 10–3.)

4. *Cervical Tilt.* The cervical tilt is designed to strengthen shoulder muscles in addition to those of the neck. First, tilt your head slowly to the left until you feel the muscles on the right side of your neck tighten. Hold this position for 3 seconds. Bring your head erect again. Repeat by tilting the head slowly to the right until you notice the tightness of the muscles on the left side of the neck. Repeat this right and left tilt three times, and gradually increase the repetitions daily until you can do twenty. (See Figure 10–4.)

Exercises for the Mid- and Lower Back

5. *Thoracic-Lumbar Lateral Flexion.* Stand erect with your feet 6 inches apart and arms at your sides. Slowly

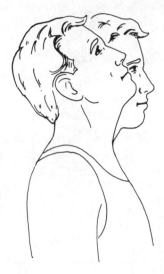

Figure 10–1. Cervical Extension.

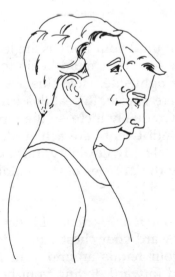

Figure 10–2. Cervical Flexion.

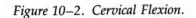

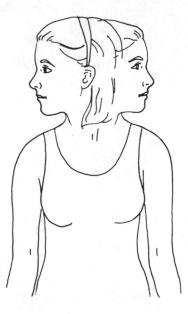

Figure 10–3. Cervical Left and Right.

lean to the left until your body is angled at approximately 20 degrees or so. You should begin to feel some muscle strain in your right side. Hold this position for 5 seconds. Slowly stand erect again. Repeat this action but bend slowly to the right. Gradually increase the repetitions of this exercise daily until twenty are achieved. In addition to increasing general body flexibility, this exercise is useful for strengthening the muscles of the middle and lower back. (See Figure 10–5.)

6. Thoracic-Lumbar Flexion. Lie flat on your back. Flex your knees toward your chest—they don't have to touch —and lock your hands around your knees. Gently roll backward and forward, letting your head move with the

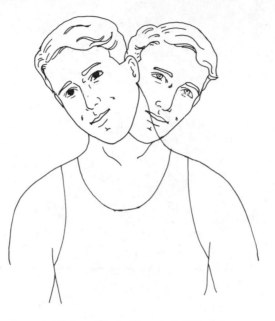

Figure 10–4. Cervical Tilt.

motion; don't try to keep your head flat on the floor. Be sure to lie on a mat, carpet, or other suitable padding, since the flexion will increase the prominence of the vertebrae. Gently roll backward and forward about five times, breathing in when you go backward and out when you go forward. Gradually increase this number daily until you can do twenty. In addition to toning up the muscles of the middle and lower back, this exercise strengthens the abdominal muscles and increases blood circulation. (See Figure 10–6.)

7. Thoracic-Lumbar Hyperextension. Lie face down on a carpet or mat with your arms outstretched in front of you. Keeping your arms straight, gently arch your back

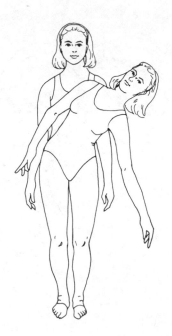

Figure 10–5. Thoracic-Lumbar Lateral Flexion.

and slowly raise your arms, head, and shoulders by tightening your back muscles. Raise yourself up, hold for a few seconds, and then lie flat and relax. This is a more strenuous exercise that will greatly increase the strength of the lower, mid, and upper back, shoulders, neck, and arms. Repeat this exercise five times, and gradually increase daily until you can do twelve. (See Figure 10–7.)

8. Thoracic-Lumbar Extension. This is one of my favorite exercises for relieving muscle tension brought about by typing for long periods of time. Kneel down on your hands and knees, with your arms supporting your shoulders. Don't worry about your feet—you can rest either on the tops of your feet or with your toes touching the ground.

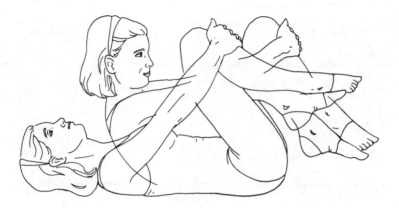

Figure 10–6. Thoracic-Lumbar Flexion.

Relax your back and slowly slump forward. Hold this position for a second or two and then slowly arch your back
to where the spine is "rounded." Roll your pelvis forward
when slumping, and backward when arching. This is a
good exercise to help you correct some of your own subluxations (you may hear several cracks or pops as you do
this exercise) and tone up the back, abdominal, and shoulder muscles. Repeat this exercise five times, and gradually
increase daily until you reach twenty. (See Figure 10–8.)

Exercise for the Abdomen

9. Abdominal Flexion. Lie flat on your back with your
arms at your sides. Anchor your feet beneath a sofa or a

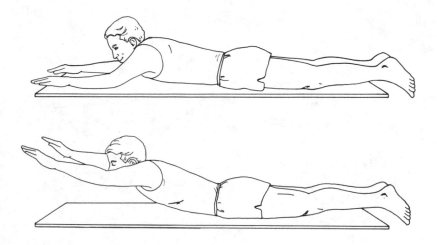

Figure 10–7. Thoracic-Lumbar Hyperextension.

friend. Gently tighten your abdominal muscles and raise your body up slowly from your waist, making sure to keep your hips on the floor. Hold for a moment, and then slowly lower yourself again to a position flat on your back. Repeat three times. Gradually increase this number daily until a series of twelve is achieved. This exercise—a variation of the sit-up—will strengthen the muscles of the abdomen, upper chest, and legs. (See Figure 10–9.)

What about Posture?

Good posture is one of the goals of chiropractic. The profession has taken a leadership role in educating parents and children on its benefits for more than fifty

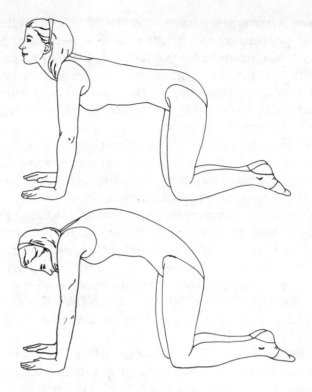

Figure 10–8. Thoracic-Lumbar Extension.

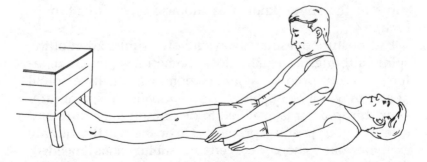

Figure 10–9. Abdominal Flexion.

years. Although we have been taught since childhood that good posture looks attractive and is necessary for coordination, chiropractors point out that it also helps keep us healthy. When the human structure is out of balance, it can produce distortions of the spine. The resulting curvature may change the position of our internal organs and cramp the lungs, stomach, and intestines, which may lead to shallow breathing, faulty digestion, and poor elimination. However, the most serious result is a vertebral subluxation, which may alter the function of various organs by affecting specific spinal nerves.

There are many reasons for poor posture. Excessive weight; negative mental attitudes; visual impairment; injury to joints, bones, or ligaments; faulty nutrition; improper sleep support (soft or sagging mattress); poorly designed chairs; vertebral subluxations—all are common contributors to poor posture. High-heeled shoes, badly designed seating in cars and trucks, and just plain laziness follow close behind.

Disturbances of body balance may show themselves in a slight tilt of the head to the right or the left, or in one shoulder (or hip) being slightly higher than the other. A sideways curve of the spine is known as *scoliosis*. There may also be an abnormal forward curve of the spine (known as cervical *lordosis* or swayback) or an abnormal backward curve of the spine (known as thoracic *kyphosis* or humpback).

Bad posture does not always involve subluxation of the spine, although it usually does. Sometimes spinal curvature may not produce a subluxation and sensitive spinal nerves may not be impaired. As a specialist in spinal care, your chiropractor is qualified to determine the nature and extent of your postural problem. He or she will thoroughly examine your spine, correct vertebral subluxations if needed, and advise how you can develop habits to promote healthy posture.

On Your Feet: Standing and Walking

Human beings are one species of a small group of animals that are bipeds. We stand erect and walk on two legs. This position gives us more agility than many other animals and enables us to lift heavy objects and enjoy greater mobility. It also creates structural demands that can become spinal disorders. For this reason, chiropractors believe learning how to stand and walk properly is important—it can help reduce the inherent gravitational and structural stresses we endure each day.

When you stand, point your toes straight ahead. Place your body weight primarily on your heels. Shift your upper chest slightly forward so that it protrudes farther out than the abdomen. Bend your knees slightly. This is not standard military posture, but an easy, relaxed position that reduces forward pull on your back and limits the possibility of strain and subluxation. If you stand for long periods of time, wear low-heeled shoes to reduce muscle strain in the lower back.

When walking, keep the toes pointed straight ahead. Keep your chest uplifted in a natural, unforced way. Be sure to lift your knees so that you are flexing the muscles of the legs and lower back. Wear low-heeled, comfortable shoes with padded soles. They keep your body closer to its natural center of gravity and reduce jarring and fatigue.

At Ease: Sitting and Sleeping

From childhood on, we are told to sit up straight to avoid spinal curvature and other results of poor posture. Slouching in a chair is a major cause of curvature of the spine. The ideal sitting position is with the shoulders slightly rounded and the knees slightly higher than the hips to prevent back strain and forward spinal curvature.

What is the "ideal chair"? According to Hyman Jampol, a physiotherapist who is director of the Beverly Palms Rehabilitation Hospital in Los Angeles, a good chair fulfills the following three requirements:

1. The seat should be inclined slightly backward for improved lower-back support.
2. The back support should be level with your shoulder blades to eliminate stress on the shoulders and neck.
3. Your thighs should be comfortably supported so that sharp edges (such as the thin seats of deck chairs) will not cut off blood circulation. If necessary, add pillows to chairs that cause back strain, or cut an inch off the rear legs of a sofa or chair that does not provide adequate low-back support. Be sensitive to your body's needs. Learn to avoid chairs or sofas that cause back pain.

Some chiropractors recommend rocking chairs because the backward and forward motion relieves pressure on the spinal muscles and prevents cramping. A small footstool is recommended for keeping the knees higher than the hips. It will take pressure off your lower back and help straighten out the lumbar area of your spine.

All chiropractors agree that a soft, sagging mattress is extremely harmful to the spine. It leads to back pain and vertebral subluxation. Since we spend approximately one-third of our lives in bed, a firm mattress with good back support is an excellent investment in health and comfort. There are many good beds available in any well-stocked furniture store. Select one that is really comfortable for you. A mattress that is too soft may allow your back to arch too much. One that is too firm may cause pain and subluxation from too much pressure. A survey by *The New York Times* found that most people preferred an "orthopedic" mattress (the King Koil® mattress has received the endorsement of the International Chiropractors Association), with water beds coming in a close second. Japanese-style cotton mattresses (futons) have gained wide popularity in recent years for their economy, comfort, and firm support.

Many chiropractors believe that the best sleep position is on your back because sleeping on the stomach arches and strains the lower back and neck. Sleeping on your side is a good idea, especially if you bring both knees up toward the chest to reduce muscle tension in the spine. Conventional pillows often contribute to neck strain, so you may wish to use a small, soft pillow or special cervical pillow that provides additional support to the neck. Many chiropractors actually sell them, although they may be found in any surgical supply store.

Gesundheit!

A strong sneeze can bring about more back injury than almost any other cause. It forces the upper part of the body to bend vigorously. Resisting the sneeze suddenly stops the upper body's natural forward motion, resulting in a powerful muscle contraction that can cause a painful subluxation. In his book *The Weekend Athlete's Way to a Pain-Free Monday*, Hyman Jampol offers the following simple advice: "To prevent injury, *bend your knees* so that you are in a half squat and do not resist the sneeze. Relax and let go."

How to Lift without Ruining Your Back

Improper lifting is a leading cause of subluxation. It strains the spinal muscles, which can pull one or more vertebrae out of alignment and cause severe pain.

We tend to place excessive weight on the lower back instead of the legs, which are designed to support far more than our body weight. We often lift with a quick, jerking motion and bring about sudden strain. Instead of holding an object close to the body, we hold it away from the natural center of gravity, throwing the entire body, especially the spine, out of balance and causing injury and pain. Learning how to lift properly is not a difficult task. The National Safety Council has recommended the following six steps (see figures 10–10, 10–11, and 10–12):

1. Your feet should be approximately 12 inches apart. One should be placed alongside the object you are lifting. The other should be located slightly behind the object. This will provide you with greater balance and stability. You will have greater strength for lifting. If you need to change positions in order to lift, move your feet instead of twisting your body.

2. Keep your back straight in a nearly vertical position. This reduces some of the pressure that builds up in the abdominal region and keeps your spine and body in proper alignment.

3. Keep your chin tucked in. This will reduce injuries to the neck and helps achieve spinal balance.

4. Grip the object with your whole hand. This prevents it from slipping, which causes a sudden shift in weight and perhaps back strain or other injury.

5. Keep your elbows and arms tucked in. Bring the object as close to your body as possible. With a closer center of gravity, lifting will be easier and your spine will remain balanced and free from strain.

6. Make sure your body weight is directly over your feet. This will help your body to balance the weight of the object and will give greater strength for lifting and carrying.

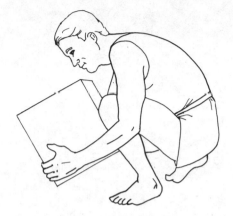

Figure 10–10. Feet parted—one alongside, one behind the object you are lifting.

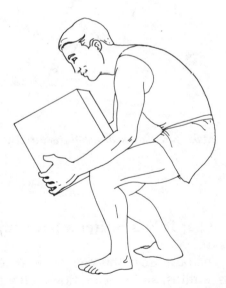

Figure 10–11. Keep your back straight, chin tucked in, and grip the object with the whole hand. Keep elbows and arms tucked in.

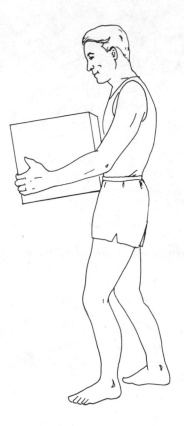

Figure 10–12. Make sure that body weight is directly over the feet.

What If You Suffer a Back Injury?

The purpose of this chapter is to help you avoid back sprains, strains, and subluxations. However, despite precautions, accidents do happen—a fall in the bathroom, reaching into a low cabinet, a sudden sneeze—that can injure the spine and cause extreme pain.

When a back injury occurs, doctors recommend that you lie down immediately in a comfortable position. Call a chiropractor and arrange to see him or her as soon as possible. Often the cause of back pain can be corrected with only one adjustment and you can be saved much pain and discomfort. Follow your chiropractor's advice about how you can facilitate recovery.

Through a program of preventive exercise, you can avoid many spinal problems that cause pain, limit activity, and open the door to ill health. Exercise can even be a pleasure. If you do every exercise described in this chapter, you do not need more than 15 or 20 minutes a day. Performed to music and in attractive surroundings, daily exercise can be a pleasure looked forward to and shared with family and friends.

Chiropractic works to preserve the integrity of our bodies and to keep us healthy, active, and strong. With a personal program of daily exercise and increased awareness of correct posture and proper lifting, you can greatly enhance the benefits of regular chiropractic care. You can learn to take greater responsibility for your health in these and other ways and to work as a partner with your chiropractor to achieve constructive survival values.

Chiropractic and Your New Health Future

The World Health Organization defines *health* as "a state of complete physical, mental, and social well-being, not just merely the absence of disease or infirmity." Most of us believe good health is our greatest treasure, but few of us can really be called healthy today. According to the newsletter *To Your Health*, all but approximately 2 percent of our nation's annual health-care bill is spent on the treatment of disease. Critics say that our health-care system is basically a "disease care" system, which works on the premise that our natural, physical state is to be sick, and the best way to health is to spend more and more money fighting disease.

The chiropractic alternative teaches that the natural state of human beings is to be healthy. Our body's inborn intelligence is perfectly designed to keep us well and active during our entire lifetime. We have a duty to take responsibility for our health by making sure our bodies function without hindrances of any kind, whether from pollution, lack of proper exercise, negative thinking, unhealthy lifestyle habits, or nerve impingement from spinal misalignments.

By taking responsibility for the causes of illness, we become aware of the dynamics of health and how we can make health a concrete reality in our lives. We make a commitment to the prevention of dis-ease rather than preserve a focus on crisis medicine. We become self-reliant rather than dependent on a health professional to periodically "fix" our symptoms. This commitment can lead to a new level of self-esteem and a joy in taking better care of ourselves and those we love.

According to a statement attributed to Thomas Edison, "The doctor of the future will give no medicine, but will interest his patients in the care of the human frame, in diet, and in the cause and prevention of disease." I believe that today's chiropractor has the potential to be the doctor of the future. Preventive health care, grounded in a Hippocratic philosophy thousands of years old, will continue to grow because it is safe, effective, and economical. As part of our future, the chiropractic alternative will lead us toward personal responsibility for our health and for the health of our children and grandchildren.

Chiropractic Colleges Worldwide

Here is a listing, as of 1990, of all the chiropractic educational institutions in the United States, Canada, England, Australia, France, and Japan.

United States

The following schools in the United States are accredited by the Council of Chiropractic Education (CCE).

Cleveland Chiropractic College
6401 Rockhill Rd.
Kansas City, MO 64131

Cleveland Chiropractic College
590 N. Vermont Ave.
Los Angeles, CA 90004

Life Chiropractic College
1269 Barclay Circ.
Marietta, GA 30063

Life Chiropractic College, West
2005 Via Barrett
P.O. Box 367
San Lorenzo, CA 94580

Logan College of Chiropractic
1851 Schoettler Rd.
P.O. Box 1065
Chesterfield, MO 63006

Los Angeles College of Chiropractic
16200 E. Amber Valley Dr.
P.O. Box 1166
Whittier, CA 90609

National College of Chiropractic
200 E. Roosevelt Rd.
Lombard, IL 60148

New York Chiropractic College
P.O. Box 167
Glen Head, NY 11545
(After September 1991 the address will be:
New York Chiropractic College
Seneca Falls, NY 13148)

Northwestern College of Chiropractic
2501 W. 84th St.
Bloomington, MN 55431

Palmer College of Chiropractic
1000 Brady St.
Davenport, IA 52803

Palmer College of Chiropractic, West
1095 Dunford Way
Sunnyvale, CA 94087

Parker College of Chiropractic
300 E. Irving Blvd.
P.O. Box 157444
Irving, TX 75015

Texas Chiropractic College
5912 Spencer Hwy.
Pasadena, TX 77505

Western States Chiropractic College
2900 N.E. 132nd St.
Portland, OR 97230

The following schools in the United States are accredited by the Straight Chiropractic Academic Standards Association (SCASA).

Pennsylvania College of Straight Chiropractic
7500 Germantown Ave.
Philadelphia, PA 19119

Sherman College of Straight Chiropractic
Springfield Rd.
P.O. Box 1452
Spartanburg, SC 29304

Southern California Chiropractic College
8420 Beverly Rd.
Pico Rivera, CA 90660

Canada

Canadian Memorial Chiropractic College
1900 Bayview Ave.
Toronto, Ontario M4G 3E6
(Status is under a reciprocal agreement with the CCE
  Canada)

England

Anglo-European College of Chiropractic
13–15 Parkwood Rd.
Bournemouth BH5 2DF

McTimoney Chiropractic School
P.O. Box 127, 14B Park End St.
Oxford OX1 1HH

Australia

Phillip Institute of Technology
School of Chiropractic
Plenty Rd.
Bundoora, Victoria 3083

The Sydney College of Chiropractic
P.O. Box 178, 4 Henson St.
Summer Hill, New South Wales 2130

France

Institut Français du Chiropractique
44 rue Duhesme
75018 Paris

Japan

Chukyo School of Chiropractic
3-12-12 Meieki, Nakamuraku
Nagoya 450

Japan School of Chiropractic
5-13-2 Ginza Chou-ku
Tokyo

Chiropractic Professional Organizations

Here is a listing, as of 1990, of the major chiropractic professional organizations for the United States, Australia, Canada, England, Europe, New Zealand, South Africa, and Japan. They are listed in order of size and prominence.

United States

American Chiropractic Association
1701 Clarendon Blvd.
Arlington, VA 22209
(Publishes *ACA Journal of Chiropractic*)

International Chiropractors Association
1110 N. Glebe Rd., Ste. 1000
Arlington, VA 22201
(Publishes *ICA International Review of Chiropractic*)

Federation of Straight Chiropractic Organizations
642 Broad St.
Clifton, NJ 07013
(Publishes *Triune*)

Australia

Australian Chiropractors' Association
459 Great Western Hwy.
Faulconbridge, New South Wales 2776

United Chiropractors Association of Australia
P.O. Box 48
Auburn, New South Wales 2114

Canada

Canadian Chiropractic Association
290 Lawrence Ave. West
Toronto, Ontario M5M 1B3

England

British Chiropractic Association
5 First Ave.
Chelmsford, Essex CM1 1RX

The Institute of Pure Chiropractic
P.O. Box 126
Oxford OX1 1UF

Europe (including Belgium, Denmark, Finland, France, West Germany, Greece, Italy, Netherlands, Norway, Spain, Sweden, and Switzerland, as well as Great Britain)

European Chiropractors Union
19 Strawberry Hill Rd.
Twickenham, Middlesex TW1 4QB, England

New Zealand

New Zealand Chiropractors' Association
DIC Building, Brandon St.
P.O. Box 2858
Wellington

South Africa

The Chiropractic Association of South Africa
701 Poynton House, Gardiner St.
Durban 4001, Natal

Japan

Japanese Chiropractic Association
3-5-9 Kita-Aoyama Minato-Ku
Tokyo 107

For a current listing of other international organizations, contact the Foundation for the Advancement of Chiropractic Tenets and Science (FACTS), 1110 N. Glebe Rd., Arlington, VA 22201.

References

Chapter 1: The Promise of Chiropractic

Louise Ackerman, "Chiropractic: An Alternative Cure for Tennis Injuries," *Tennis*, February 1987, pp. 105–106.

Marcus Bach, *The Chiropractic Story* (Los Angeles: DeVorss, 1968).

G. Bery, et al., "Low Back Pain During Pregnancy," *Obstetrics Gynecology*, 1988, 71: pp. 71–75.

T. W. Bunch and G. G. Hunder, "Ankylosing Spondylitis and Primary Hyperparathyroidism," *Journal of the American Medical Association*, 27 August 1973, pp. 1108–1109.

Arno Burnier, "The Birth of Subluxations," *Today's Chiropractic*, September/October 1985, pp. 13, 30.

William Burrows, *Textbook of Microbiology* (Philadelphia: Saunders, 1959).

The Canadian Family Physician, July 1969, pp. 35–39.

The Canadian Family Physician, 1985, Vol. 3, pp. 535–540.

E. Celander, A.J. Koenig, D.R. Celander, "Effect of Osteopathic Manipulative Therapy on Autonomic Tone," *Journal of the American Osteopathic Association*, May 1968.

"Changes in the Cervical Spine," *Manuelle Medizine*, 6 (1973).

"Leading by Example," *Chiropractic Achievers*, March/April 1989, pp. 25–28.

"Chiropractic Effectiveness with Emotional, Learning, and Behavioral Impairments," *International Review of Chiropractic*, November 1975.

Chiropractic State of the Art (Des Moines: American Chiropractic Association, October 1979).

Chiropractic State of the Art 1989–1990 (Arlington, Va.: American Chiropractic Association, 1989).

Commission of Inquiry into Chiropractic, *Chiropractic in New Zealand* (Wellington: Government Printer, 1979).

Althea Courtenay, *Chiropractic for Everyone* (London: Penguin Books, 1987).

A. B. Coyer and I. H. M. Curwen, "Low Back Pain Treated by

Manipulation," *British Medical Journal*, 19 March 1955, pp. 705–707.

L. Crispini and E. Mantero, "Static Alterations of the Pelvic, Sacral Lumber Area Due to Pregnancy: Chiropractic Treatment," in *Chiropractic: Interprofessional Research*, J. Mazzarelli, ed. (Torino: Edizioni Minerva Medica, 1983), pp. 59–68.

James Cyriax, *Treatment by Manipulation and Massage* (London: Paul B. Hoeber, 1979).

David Davis, "Spinal Nerve Root Pain Simulating Coronary Occlusion," *American Heart Journal*, January 1948, pp. 70–80.

Laurence De Mann, "What Cracks While Cracking," *Dancemagazine*, September 1984.

D. J. Duffy, *A Study of Wisconsin Back Injury Cases* (Madison: University of Wisconsin, August 1978).

11 Common Questions About Chiropractic (Washington: The International Chiropractors Association, no date).

Frank R. Ford, "Syncope, Vertigo, Vision Problems Resulting from Obstruction," *Bulletin of Johns Hopkins Hospital*, 91 (1952), pp. 168–173.

E. D. Gardner, *Fundamentals of Neurology* (Philadelphia: W. B. Saunders, 1968).

J. J. Gartland, "Barre Lieau Syndrome," *Foundations of Orthopedics* (Philadelphia: W. B. Saunders, Inc., 1965).

K. Gundrum, "Whiplash Injuries to the Ear," *International Record of Medicine and G.P. Clinics*, January 1956, pp. 21–25.

J. M. Hoag, "Musculoskeletal Involvement in Chronic Lung Disease," *Journal of the American Osteopathic Association*, April 1972, pp. 57–65.

Robin Hood, "Blood Pressure," *The Digest of Chiropractic Economics*, May/June 1974, pp. 36–38.

A. J. Josey and F. Murphey, "Ruptured Intervertebral Disk Simulating Angina Pectoris," *Journal of the American Medical Association*, 15 June 1946, pp. 581–587.

Journal of the American Medical Association, 19 April 1971, p. 520.

Marjorie R. Johnson, et al., "Treatment and Cost of Back or Neck Injury—A Literature Review," *Research Forum*, Spring 1985, pp. 68–78.

Blair Justice, *Who Gets Sick* (Los Angeles: Jeremy P. Tarcher, 1988).

Barbara Kelves, "The Chiropractor," *Esquire*, April 1984, pp. 18, 20.

Tedd Koren, "Cancer and Chiropractic," *International Review of Chiropractic*, September 1977.

M. LaBan, et al., "Sexual Impotence in Men Having Low Back Syndrome," *Archives of Physical Medicine and Rehabilitation*, November 1966, pp. 715–723.

Robert A. Leach, *The Chiropractic Theories*, 2nd ed. (Baltimore: Williams and Wilkins, 1986).

K. Lewit, *Manual Therapy* ()Leipzig: J. A. Barth, 1973).

J. G. Love and J. L. Emmet, "Asymptomatic Protruded Lumbar Disc as a Cause of Urinary Retention," *Mayo Clinic Proceedings*, May 1967, pp. 249–257.

Medical Journal of Australia, 14 January 1967, pp. 78–79.

John McM. Mennell, *Back Pain* (Boston: Little Brown, 1960).

Tom O'Connor with Ahmed Gonzalez-Nunez, *Living with AIDS* (San Francisco: Corwin Publishers, 1987).

Daniel O'Donovan, "Possible Significance of Scoliosis of the Spine in the Causation of Asthma and Allied Allergic Conditions," *Annals of Allergy*, March-April 1951, pp. 184–189.

G. B. Parker, et al., "A Controlled Trial of Cervical Manipulation for Migraine," *Australia and New Zealand Journal of Medicine*, December 1978, pp. 589–593.

"Pathogenic Importance of the Thoracic Portion of the Vertebral Column," *Arch. Orthop. Unfall. Chir.*, 19, No. 6, 1958.

Margaret Pierpoint, "What Chiropractic Can Do for the Dancer," *Dancemagazine*, January 1980, pp. 88–89.

Robb Russell, "Cost-Effective Care of Industrial Back Injury," *Journal of Chiropractic*, May 1985, pp. 40 41.

R. C. Schafer, *Chiropractic Management of Sports and Recreational Injuries*, 2nd ed. (Baltimore: Williams and Wilkins, 1986).

Herman S. Schwartz, ed., *Mental Health and Chiropractic* (New Hyde Park, N.Y.: Sessions Publishers, 1973).

Jason Serinus, ed., *Psychoimmunity and the Healing Process* (Berkeley, Calif.: Celestial Arts, 1986).

Spears Hospital News, May-December 1979 (various issues).

"Spinal Manipulation," *The Canadian Family Physician*, July 1969.

Louis Sportelli, *Introduction to Chiropractic*, 9th ed. (Palmerton, Pa.: Practice Makers Productions Inc., 1988).

"The Good Hands Man," *Sports Illustrated*, 16 July 1979.

"Symposium: Indications for and Techniques of Spinal Manipulation," *Medical Journal of Australia*, 28 September 1968, pp. 555–558.

Time, 19 March 1973, p. 65.

Abraham Towbin, "Latent Spinal Cord and Brain Stem Injury in Newborn Infants," *Developmental Medicine and Child Neurology*, 11 (1969), pp. 54–68.

Abraham Towbin, "Neonatal CNS Damage," *American Journal of Diseases of Children*, June 1970, pp. 531–532.

"The Treatment of Subluxation Headaches," *Therapie Genewart* (Heft 5, 1951), pp. 175–179.

Neville T. Ussher, "Spinal Curvatures—Visceral Disturbances in Relation Thereto," *California and Western Medicine*, June 1933.

Chester A. Wilk, *Chiropractic Speaks Out* (Park Ridge, Ill.: Wilk Publishing Co., 1976).

M. E. Williamson, "Thyroid Dysfunction and Somatic Reflection," *Journal of the American Osteopathic Association*, March 1973, pp. 731–737.

T. J. Wilmont, "Cervical Vertigo," *The Lancet*, 7 January 1956, p. 52.

P. T. Wilson, *The Osteopathic Treatment of Asthma*, July 1946.

A. H. Wolf, "Osteopathic Manipulative Procedure in Disorders of the Eye," *Yearbook of the Academy of Applied Osteopathy*, 1970.

S. S. Yang, et al., "Upper Cervical Myelopathy in Achondroplasia," *American Journal of Clinical Pathology*, July 1977, pp. 68–72.

Chapter 2: Chiropractic: What It Is and What It's Not

Fred H. Barge, *Life Without Fear* (Eldridge, Ia.: Bawden Bros. Inc., 1987).

Brief to the Royal Commission on Health Services (Toronto: Canadian Chiropractic Association, May 1962).

Joseph A. Califano, Jr., "Billions Blown on Health," *The New York Times*, 12 April 1989.

Chiropractic State of the Art 1989–1990.

Marggi Dobos, ed., *C.A.S.E. History* (Spartanburg, S.C.: Sherman College of Straight Chiropractic, 1985).

Cathy M. Garris, "Are D.O.'s Real Doctors?" *Journal of the Medical Association of Georgia*, March 1985, pp. 162–163.

Reginald R. Gold, *The Triune of Life* (Davenport, Ia.: International Chiropractors Association, 1966).

Ann Hill, ed., *A Visual Encyclopedia of Unconventional Medicine* (New York: Crown Publishers, 1979).

ICA Position Statement (Washington: International Chiropractors Association, August 1979).

Indexed Synopsis of ACA Policies on Public Health and Related Matters (Arlington, Va.: The American Chiropractic Association, 1988).

Brian Inglis, *The Case for Unorthodox Medicine* (New York: G. P. Putnam's Sons, 1965).

Blair Justice, *Who Gets Sick* (Los Angeles: Jeremy P. Tarcher, 1988).

Peter Marsh, "Prescribing All the Way to the Bank," *New Scientist*, 18 November 1989, pp. 50–55.

Eric Martin, ed., *Hazards of Medication* (New York: Lippincott, 1971).

Joseph E. Maynard, *Healing Hands* (Freeport, N.Y.: Jonorm Publishing, 1959).

Simon Mills and S. J. Finaldo, *Alternatives in Healing* (New York: New American Library, 1989).

The New York Times, 25 November 1979, section 4, p. 7.

Gary Null, "Prescription for Disaster," *Penthouse*, September 1985.

Vincent C. Nwuga, *Manipulation of the Spine* (Baltimore: Williams and Wilkins, 1976).

"The Osteopathic School of Medicine," *University of Toronto Medical Journal*, February 1961.

B. J. Palmer, *The Science of Chiropractic*, Vol. 1, 4th ed. (Davenport: Palmer School of Chiropractic, 1920).

B. J. Palmer, *Up from Below the Bottom* (Davenport: Chiropractic Fountain Head, 1950).

D. D. Palmer, *The Science, Art and Philosophy of Chiropractic* (Portland: Portland Printing House Co., 1910).

Maud Russel, ed., "Acupuncture: Some Basic Facts," *Far East Reporter*, March 1972, pp. 14–16, 86–104, 106.

R. C. Schafer, *Basic Chiropractic Paraprofessional Manual* (Des Moines: American Chiropractic Association, 1978).

R. C. Schafer, *Chiropractic Health Care* (Des Moines: The Foundation for Chiropractic Education and Research, 1978).

Science, 13 September 1974, p. 923.

Robert Shestack, *Handbook of Physical Therapy*, 3rd. ed. (New York: Springer Publishing Co., 1977).

Virgil V. Strang, *Essential Principles of Chiropractic* (Davenport: Palmer College of Chiropractic, 1984).

Touch for Health Newsletter, August 1979, pp. 1–2.

Triune, Summer 1987; Winter 1988–1989.

U.S. Bureau of the Census, *Statistical Abstract of the United States: 1989* (Washington: U.S. Government Printing Office, 1989).

Fu Wei-Kang, *The Story of Chinese Acupuncture and Moxibustion* (Beijing: Foreign Language Press, 1975).

Andrew Weil, *Health and Healing* (Boston: Houghton Mifflin Co., 1983).

H. J. Weiss, "Aspirin—A Dangerous Drug," *Journal of the American Medical Association*, 26 August 1974, pp. 1221–1222.

Chapter 3: Chiropractic's Controversial History

Francis Adams, trans., *The Genuine Works of Hippocrates*, Vol. 2 (New York: William Wood & Co., 1886).

AMA Principles of Medical Ethics, 1955 ed., chap. 2, sec. 1.

Marcus Bach, *The Chiropractic Story*.

Fred H. Barge, *Life Without Fear*.

J. H. Breasted, trans., *The Edwin Smith Surgical Papyrus*, Vol. 1 (Chicago: University of Chicago Press, 1930).

"Chiropractic," *University of Toronto Journal of Medicine*, February 1961.

"Chiropractic: Its History and Challenge to Medicine," *The Pharos*, April 1978.

Letter from J. W. Colgan, M.D., to Nicholas W. VanLeeuwen, M.D., August 23, 1963.

FACTS Bulletin, Foundation for the Advancement of Chiropractic Tenets and Science and the International Chiropractors Association, Vol. 2, 1986–1987.

Finally After 11 Years the Federal Court in Chicago, Illinois Found the American Medical Association Guilty!!! (Huntington Beach, Calif.: Motion Palpation Institute, 1987).

Joseph Garland, *The Story of Medicine* (Boston: Houghton Mifflin, 1949).

Russell W. Gibbons, *Chiropractic History: Lost, Strayed or Stolen* (Davenport: Palmer College Student Council, January 1976).

Murray Goldstein, ed., *The Research Status of Spinal Manipulative Medicine* (Bethesda, Md.: U.S. Department of Health, Education and Welfare, 1975).

Scott Haldeman, ed., *Modern Developments in the Principles and Practice of Chiropractic* (Norwalk, Conn.: Appleton Century Crofts, 1980), pp. 3–24, 25–41.

Brian Inglis, *The Book of the Back*. (New York: Hearst Books, 1978).

F. Le Corre, "Historique des Manipulations Vertebrales," *Les Cahiers de College de Medecine des Hospitaux de Paris*, September 1968.

Letter from D. S. Masland, M.D., to guidance counselors in Pennsylvania High Schools and Colleges, January 23, 1976.

Joseph E. Maynard, *Healing Hands*.

The New York Times, 31 August 1987, p. 1.

B. J. Palmer, *History in the Making* (Davenport: Chiropractic Fountain Head, 1957).

D. D. Palmer, *The Science, Art and Philosophy of Chiropractic*.

D. D. Palmer, *Three Generations* (Davenport: Palmer College of Chiropractic, 1967).

"Quiet AMA Referral Revision Appears to Affect Chiropractors," *International Review of Chiropractic*, May 1977.

"Radiologists Vow Battle Against Chiropractic, FTC," *American Medical News*, 28 April 1978.

Arthur Scofield, *Chiropractice* (Wellingborough, U.K.: Thorsons Publishers, 1968).

J. E. Stolfi, "AMA Surrenders to Chiropractors," *New York State Journal of Medicine*, April 1979, pp. 782–787.

"Suit Alleges Broad Conspiracy Intended to Stop Chiropractic," *Hospitals*, 1 August 1979, p. 18.

Triune, Spring 1988, p. 8.

Walter I. Wardwell, "The Future of Chiropractic," *The New England Journal of Medicine*, 20 March 1980.

Chester A. Wilk, *Chiropractic Speaks Out*.

Memorandum from R. A. Youngerman to H. D. Taylor (Director, Dept. of Investigation, AMA), 21 September 1967.

Chapter 4: How Chiropractic Works: The Education of the Patient

Darald Bolin, *The Philosophy of Chiropractic* (Philadelphia: Dorrance, 1974).

Arno Burnier, "The End of Controversy," *Today's Chiropractic*, July/August 1985, p. 17.

Walter B. Cannon, *The Wisdom of the Body* (New York: W.W. Norton, 1963).

E. Clarke and C. D. O'Malley, *The Human Brain and Spinal Cord* (Berkeley: University of California Press, 1968).

Frank DeGiacomo, *Man's Greatest Gift to Man . . . Chiropractic* (Old Bethpage, N.Y.: LSR Learning Associates, 1978).

Digest of Chiropractic Economics, November/December 1986, pp. 58, 60–61.

Julius Dintenfass, *Chiropractic: A Modern Way to Health* (New York: Pyramid Books, 1973).

Robert Dishman, "Review of the Literature Supplying a Scientific Basis for the Chiropractic Subluxation Complex," *Journal of Manipulative and Physiological Therapeutics,* September 1985, pp. 163–174.

Donald Epstein, "Chiropractic Principles and Practice in the Network Model," *Beacon,* April 1987, p. 4.

Donald Epstein, "The Stress Connection: Gauging the Role of The Nervous System," *Today's Chiropractic,* December 1986/January 1987, pp. 15–17.

FSCO (Lawrence, Kan.: Federation of Straight Chiropractic Organizations, 1979).

Murray Goldstein, ed., *The Research Status of Spinal Manipulative Therapy* (Bethesda, Md.: U.S. Dept. of Health, Education and Welfare, 1975).

Scott Haldeman, *International Review of Chiropractic,* 28(10): 14–15, 26–27, 1973.

A. E. Homewood, *The Neurodynamics of the Vertebral Subluxation* (St. Petersburg, Fla.: Valkyrie Press, 1977).

ICA Policy Statement: Definition of Subluxation (Washington, D.C.: International Chiropractors Association, January 1988).

Brian Inglis, *The Book of the Back.*

Journal of Manipulative and Physiological Therapeutics, March 1982, pp. 1–3.

Blair Justice, *Who Gets Sick.*

I. M. Korr, "Osteopathic Research, Why, What, Whither?" *Journal of the American Osteopathic Association* 56(5): 275–285, 1957.

Donald Law, *The Guide to Alternative Medicine* (New York: Hippocrene Books, 1975).

Robert A. Leach, *The Chiropractic Theories.*

S. M. Levy, ed., *Biological Mediators of Behavior and Disease: Neoplasma* (New York: Elsevier, 1982).

D. D. Palmer, *The Science, Art and Philosophy of Chiropractic.*

T. P. Pick and R. Howdon, *Gray's Anatomy* (New York: Bounty Books, 1977).

R. C. Schafer, *Chiropractic Health Care.*

R. C. Schafer, *Chiropractic Management of Sports and Recreational Injuries.*

Herman Schwartz, *Mental Health and Chiropractic.*

Louis Sportelli, *Introduction to Chiropractic.*

Ralph W. Stephenson, Chiropractic Text Book (Davenport: Palmer School of Chiropractic, 1926).

Virgil V. Strang, *Essential Principles of Chiropractic.*

J. P. Warbasse, "Dislocations of Cervical Vertebrae," *American Journal of Surgery,* March 1909, pp. 105–107.

J. P. Warbasse, *Surgical Treatment*, Vol. 1 (Philadelphia: W. B. Saunders, 1920).
Chester A. Wilk, *Chiropractic Speaks Out*.

Chapter 5: The Education of the Chiropractor

Arturo Castiglioni, *A History of Medicine* (New York: Alfred A. Knopf, 1947).
Chiropractic State of the Art 1988–1989.
Council on Chiropractic Education, *1988 Report* (Des Moines: Council of Chiropractic Education, 1988).
Abraham Flexner, *Medical Education in the United States and Canada* (New York: The Carnegie Foundation for the Advancement of Technology, 1910).
FSCO President's Update, May/June 1988.
International Review of Chiropractic, April/June 1979, p. 36.
Medical Economics, 27 May 1985, pp. 81–85; 4 January 1988, pp. 58–66.
1989 Examination Information (Greeley, Co.: National Board of Chiropractic Examiners, 1988).
Official Directory of Chiropractic and Basic Science Examining Boards with Licensure and Practice Statistics (Glendale, Calif.: Federation of Chiropractic Licensing Boards, 1979).
R. C. Schafer, *Chiropractic Health Care*.
Chester A. Wilk, *Chiropractic Speaks Out*.

Chapter 6: Choosing the Right Chiropractor

Fred H. Barge, "A Solution to Pollution," *The American Chiropractor*, June 1989.
The Cactus Flower, April 1979, pp. 6–7.
Charter Provisions and Bylaws (Arlington, Va.: American Chiropractic Association, 1988).
"Chiropractic Comes of Age," *Family Health*, December 1978.
The Chiropractic Journal, April 1989, pp. 1, 7; May 1989, p. 14.
Chiropractic White Paper (Des Moines: American Chiropractic Association; Davenport: International Chiropractors Association; Cheyenne, Wyo.: Council of State Chiropractic Licensing Boards, May 1969).
P. D. Cleary, "Chiropractic Use: A Test of Several Hypotheses," *American Journal of Public Health*, July 1982, pp. 727–729.

"Controversy Continued," *The American Chiropractor*, December 1979.
Frank DeGiacomo, *Man's Greatest Gift*.
Scott Haldeman, ed., *Principles and Practice of Chiropractic*, pp. 25–41.
Samuel Homola, *Bonesetting, Chiropractic and Cultism* (Panama City, Fla.: Critique Books, 1963).
Impulse, June 1979, pp. 2–3, 8–9.
Karl Kranz, "Hospital Access," *ICA Review of Chiropractic*, November/December 1987, pp. 27–33.
Medical World News, 11 December 1978, pp. 57–72.
B. J. Palmer, *The Science of Chiropractic*.
D. D. Palmer, *The Science, Art and Philosophy of Chiropratic*.
Pennsylvania Medicine, May 1979, pp. 54–56.
R. C. Schafer, *Chiropractic Health Care*.
Rose Spector, "Guide to New York's Hottest Holistic Chiropractors," *Whole Life*, January/February 1989, pp. 40–41.
"The Straights versus the Chiropractors," *International Review of Chiropractic*, October/December 1979.
Virgil V. Strang, *Essential Principles of Chiropractic*.
Triune, Winter/Spring 1987, pp. 5–6, 9.
Chester A. Wilk, *Chiropractic Speaks Out*.

Chapter 7: A Visit to a Chiropractor: What to Expect

The Chiropractic Journal, March 1989, pp. 13, 18.
Chiropractic State of the Art 1989–1990, pp. 48–49.
"Chiropractors: Healers or Quacks?" *Pennsylvania Medicine*, May 1976.
"Chiropractors Pushing for a Place on the Health Care Team," *Medical World News*, 11 December 1978.
Frank DeGiacomo, *Man's Greatest Gift*.
Scott Haldeman, *Principles and Practice of Chiropractic*, pp. 231–261.
Samuel Homola, *Bonesetting*.
Journal of Clinical Chiropractic, Vol. 2, No. 4, 1968.
R. L. Kane, et al., "Manipulating the Patient: A Comparison of the Effectiveness of Physician and Chiropractic Care," *The Lancet*, 29 June 1974, pp. 1333–1336.
V. F. Logan and F. M. Murray, *Textbook of Logan Basic Methods* (Chesterfield, Mo.: LBM Inc., 1978).

Eva Maria Norlyk, "Beyond Bones: A New Chiropractic System Strives to Align Body and Soul," *East West*, December 1989, p. 26.

G. J. Rockley and M. G. Rockley, "Breakthroughs in Computer-Assisted Thermal Imagers," *Today's Chiropractic*, January/February 1989, pp. 55–57.

Chapter 8: Chiropractic Survival Values

Fred H. Barge, *Life Without Fear*.

Herbert Bensen, *The Relaxation Response* (New York: Avon Books, 1976).

Norman Cousins, *Anatomy of an Illness* (New York: W.W. Norton, 1979).

Donald Epstein, "The Spinal Meningeal Functional Unit Tension and Stress Adaptation," *The Digest of Chiropractic Economics*, November/December 1986.

Blair Justice, *Who Gets Sick*.

Arthur Kaslow and Richard Miles, *Freedom from Chronic Disease* (Los Angeles: Jeremy P. Tarcher, 1979).

Yogi Ramacharaka, *Science of Breath* (Chicago: Yogi Publication Society, 1905).

H. Saraydarian, *The Science of Meditation* (Agoura, Calif.: The Aquarian Educational Group, 1971).

Hans Selye, *The Stress of Life* (New York: McGraw Hill, 1976).

Hans Selye, *Stress Without Distress* (New York: Signet, 1975).

O. Carl Simonton, Stephanie Matthews-Simonton, and James Creighton, *Getting Well Again* (Los Angeles: Jeremy P. Tarcher, 1978).

Ralph W. Stephenson, *Chiropractic Text Book*.

Ernest Wood, *Concentration: An Approach to Meditation* (Wheaton, Ill.: Quest Books, 1968).

Chapter 9: Eating for Life and Spinal Health

Nathaniel Altman, *Eating for Life* (New York: Vegetus Publications, 1984).

Nathaniel Altman, *Total Vegetarian Cooking* (New Canaan, Conn.: Keats Publishing, 1981).

M. S. Ansari, ed., *Symposium on Nutrition and Chiropractic Pro-*

ceedings (Davenport: Board of Nutrition, Palmer College of Chiropractic, 1986).

Rudolph Ballantine, *Diet & Nutrition* (Honesdale, Pa.: The Himalayan International Institute, 1978).

Chiropractic State of the Art 1989–1990, p. 17.

"Chiropractors," *Gary Null's Natural Living Newsletter*, Vol. 1, No. 5, pp. 1–8.

Dietary Guidelines for Americans, Home and Garden Bulletin no. 232, United States Department of Agriculture (Washington, D.C.: U. S. Government Printing Office, 1985).

"Nutrition and Chiropractic," *Bestways*, August 1979.

B. J. Palmer, *Up from Below the Bottom*, p. 568.

Louis Sportelli, *Introduction to Chiropractic*, p. 17.

Statistical Abstract of the United States: 1989, p. 105.

Ralph W. Stephenson, *Chiropractic Text Book*, pp. 127–128.

To Your Health, Fall 1987.

Chapter 10: Staying in Shape: Exercise for a Healthy Spine

Glenn D. Braatz, *Spine Care I & II* (Minneapolis: Spinal Care Publishings, 1962, 1976).

Hyman Jampol, *The Weekend Athlete's Way to a Pain-Free Monday* (Los Angeles: Jeremy P. Tarcher, 1978).

Thomas Pipes and Paul Vodak, *The Pipes Fitness Test and Prescription* (Los Angeles: Jeremy P. Tarcher, 1978).

Anne Kent Rush, *The Back Book* (Berkeley and New York: Moon Books/Summit Books, 1979).

Epilogue

Taber's Cyclopedic Medical Dictionary (Philadelphia: F.A. Davis Co., 1977).

To Your Health, Spring 1987, p. 1.

Glossary

The following glossary is intended to offer simple definitions of many terms related to chiropractic.

Adjustment. The chiropractic procedure of correcting or realigning misplaced vertebrae (*see* Subluxation) in order to reduce nerve interference. Using the bony processes of the vertebra, it is mostly characterized by a dynamic thrust of controlled amplitude. The force and velocity may vary from barely a light touch to a forceful, high-velocity thrust.

Analysis. The term used by chiropractors to denote their findings after checking the spine for any nerve interference or pressure due to subluxation.

Atlas. The first or topmost vertebra of the cervical spine, which supports the skull and allows us to nod our heads. The atlas is more subject to misalignment than most of the other vertebrae of the spine.

Autonomic nervous system. The part of the nervous system regulating involuntary responses of the body, especially those concerned with digestion, reproduction, elimination, and circulation.

Axis. The second vertebra of the cervical spine, located just below the atlas.

Central nervous system. The part of the nervous system comprised of the brain, the spinal cord, and portions of spinal nerves still encased within the vertebra. It helps the body adapt to its external environment and involves such processes as sensing and locomotion.

Cervical (ser-vi-cal). The neck region, which encompasses the first seven vertebrae of the spine.

Chiropractic. That science which concerns itself with the relationship between structure (primarily the spine) and function (primarily the nervous system) of the human body, as that relationship may affect the restoration and preservation of health. It denotes a system of adjusting the misalignments of the spine for the correction of the cause of dis-ease.

Chiropractor. A specially trained health professional who adjusts the joints, particularly the spine, mostly by hand with the primary aim of removing nerve interference.

Coccyx (kok-siks). A small triangular bone at the lower end of the spine, formed by four fused rudimentary vertebrae. It is commonly called the *tailbone*.

Correction. A term used to denote an adjustment of the spine.

Curvature. An abnormal curving of the spine.

Curve. Any one of the normal front-to-back curves of the spine, as opposed to *curvature*. Maintenance of normal curves should begin during childhood.

Disc. A small pad of cartilage. It is the "shock absorber" located between each vertebra and the next. It provides cushioning and flexibility of the spine and helps to hold the vertebrae in place.

Dis-ease. Lack of ease, or disorder within the body, which leads to impairment of bodily health and to illness. It is "that condition which allows disease to exist" and is caused by misaligned vertebrae placing pressure on spinal nerves.

Dorsal. A term biologically associated with a region of the spine containing the next twelve vertebrae below the cervical region. This area is also known as the *midback* or *thoracic* region.

Educated intelligence. Acquired knowledge based wholly on training or experience.

Hip bone. Either of the two large bones forming the sides of the pelvis. An imbalance of either of these bones may contribute to subluxation.

Iatrogenic (i-at-ro-*jen*-ic) disease. Any disease caused by drugs or medical therapy.

Ilium (*il*-e-um). The wide, upper crest of each half of the pelvis.

Innate intelligence. The inborn wisdom of the human body, which maintains and coordinates the body functions by way of the nervous system.

Intervertebral foramen (in-ter-*ver*-te-bral fo-*ra*-men). An opening located between the vertebrae of the spine that provides a passageway for nerves and blood vessels between the spinal cord and the rest of the body. Misalignment of the vertebrae can change the size and shape of this opening, causing pressure and irritation to nerves. One of the main goals of chiropractic is to keep this passageway open. Plural: intervertebral foramina.

Ischium (*is*-ke-um). The lower part of the hip bone; the area upon which we sit.

Kyphosis (ky-*fo*-sis). An abnormal backward curve of the spine. If occurring in the thoracic area, it is called *humpback*.

Lordosis (lor-*do*-sis). An abnormal forward curve of the spine. If occurring in the lumbar area, it is called *swayback*.

Lumbar. An area comprising the lower part of the spine located below the thoracic area and above the sacrum. The lumbar area of the spine normally contains five vertebrae.

This region is also known as the *lower back*, where subluxations often occur.

Manipulation. A generalized manual procedure that resets bones, increases the range of movement, and realigns joint structure in order to stimulate or inhibit body functions.

Mental impulses. Impulses that are created in the brain and directed over the entire nervous system to control cell function.

Misalignment. A term used to denote a vertebra out of normal position.

Nerve. A highly sensitive cordlike fiber that carries impulses between the central nervous system and the body organs and tissues.

Nerve pressure. Abnormal pressure on the nervous system due to one or more bones of the spine being out of place. Pressure on nerves (*neurothlipsis*) causes loss of normal function and can bring pain, paralysis, and reduced efficiency of a particular organ or tissue.

Nervous system. The "key" system that controls and coordinates all organs and structures of the human body. It consists of the brain, spinal cord, and a vast network of other nerves that extend to every part of the body. The condition of the nervous system determines to a large degree our state of health. *See* Autonomic Nervous System, Central Nervous System, Parasympathetic Nervous System, and Sympathetic Nervous System.

Neurothlipsis (nu-ro-*thlip*-sis). From the Greek words *neuron* ("nerve") and *thlipsis* ("pressure"). The principal goal of chiropractic is to eliminate neurothlipsis and ensure a continued and uninterrupted flow of normal nerve impulses between the brain and every cell in the body.

Occiput (ok-si-put). Also known as the *occipital bone*, it is situated at the back part of the base of the skull, resting on the topmost vertebra of the spine. The spinal cord passes through an opening in the occiput (called the *foramen magnum*) and down through the spinal column.

Pain. A signal with which the body reacts in self-defense to protect its mechanical integrity. Regis, a pupil of Descartes, wrote: "The great engineer of the universe has made man as perfectly as he could make him, and could not have invented a better device for his maintenance than to provide him with a sense of pain."

Parasympathetic nervous system. That part of the autonomic nervous system whose functions include the constriction of the pupils, dilation of blood vessels, slowing of the heart, increased activity of the glands, and operation of the digestive and reproductive organs.

Sacrum (say-krum). A triangular-shaped bone that forms part of the base of the spine. Composed of five segments at birth, it fuses into one bone during early childhood.

Scoliosis (sko-li-o-sis). A lateral or sideways curvature of the spine.

Spinal column. The main supporting structure of the human body, consisting of twenty-four vertebrae as well as the sacrum and coccyx.

Spinal cord. The main cable of nerves within the spinal column extending downward from the brain. The spinal nerves branch out from the spinal cord and unite the brain with all body organs and tissues.

Spinous process. This is the part of each vertebra that we can see and feel protruding along the back. It is often used by a chiropractor to help determine misalignment.

Spur. An abnormal bony projection from a vertebra or another bone.

Subluxation (sub-luk-*sa*-shun). A condition in which one or more vertebrae are out of alignment to such an extent that a nerve is impinged and the normal transmission of nerve energy is obstructed. The main goal of a chiropractor is to correct subluxations.

Sympathetic nervous system. That part of the autonomic nervous system made of two cords on either side of the spinal column, which is connected by nerve fibers to blood vessels, glands, and muscles. It works opposite the parasympathetic nervous system to accelerate the heart, decrease activity of the glands, and so on.

Thoracic (thor-*as*-ik). Also known as *dorsal*, it is a term used to describe each of the twelve vertebrae located between the neck (cervical area) and the small of the back (lumbar area).

Transverse process. A projection on each side of a vertebra for the attachment of muscles and ligaments.

Vertebra (*ver*-te-brah). A single segment or bone of the spine. Plural: vertebrae.

Recommended Reading

Healthy Intentions and Stress Management

Concentration: An Approach to Meditation. Ernest Wood. Wheaton, Ill.: Quest Books, 1968. A respected classic on mind control and meditation.

Getting Well Again. O. Carl Simonton, M.D., Stephanie Matthews-Simonton, and James Creighton. Los Angeles: Jeremy P. Tarcher, 1978. Also available from Bantam Books. A book primarily for cancer patients, but an excellent guide toward reclaiming and keeping our health. A very important book.

Guide to Yoga Meditation. Richard Hittleman. New York: Bantam Books, 1969. An excellent beginner's guide to meditation.

How to Meditate. Lawrence LeShan. New York: Bantam Books, 1975.

Love Your Disease. John Harrison, M.D. Santa Monica, Calif.: Hay House, 1989. How accident and illness can bring about long-term healing and self-understanding.

Meditation: A Practical Study. Adelaide Gardner. Wheaton, Ill.: Quest Books, 1968.

The Relaxation Response. Herbert Bensen, M.D. New York: Avon, 1972. Simple meditative techniques to manage anxiety and stress.

Stress Management. Edward A. Charlesworth and Ronald G. Nathan. New York: Ballantine, 1984.

Stress Without Distress. Hans Selye, M.D. New York: Signet, 1975. Discusses how to make stress work for you.

Who Gets Sick. Blair Justice, Ph.D. Los Angeles: Jeremy P. Tarcher, 1988. Addresses how beliefs, moods, and thoughts affect our health.

Diet and Nutrition

The Complete Guide to Health and Nutrition. Gary Null. New York: Delta, 1984. A well-documented book by the noted authority on natural living.

Diet & Nutrition. Rudolph Ballantine, M.D. Honesdale, Pa.: The Himalayan International Institute, 1978.

Diet for a New America. John Robbins. Walpole, N.H.: Stillpoint Publishing, 1987. How our food choices affect both personal health and global ecology. Highly recommended.

Food and Healing. Annemarie Colbin. New York: Ballantine, 1986. A well-researched guide to nutrition and diet.

Jane Brody's Good Food Book and *Jane Brody's Nutrition Book.* New York: Bantam Books, 1982. Two excellent guides by the *New York Times* columnist.

Laurel's Kitchen. Laurel Robertson, Carol Flinders, and Bronwen Godfrey. New York: Bantam Books, 1976. An outstanding guide to healthy vegetarian eating. Includes hundreds of recipes.

Exercise for a Healthy Spine

Bikram's Beginning Yoga Class. Bikram Choudhury with Bonnie Jones Reynolds. Los Angeles: Jeremy P. Tarcher, 1978. An excellent yoga book written with humor and charm.

Bodywise. Joseph Heller and William A. Henkin. Los Angeles: Jeremy P. Tarcher, 1986. A book on the philosophy and practice of healthy exercise and movement.

The Complete Illustrated Book of Yoga. Swami Vishnudevananda. New York: Pocket Books, 1972. A compete yoga book for the beginning or advanced student.

Low Impact Aerobics. Kathryn Lane. New York: Crown, 1988. A guide to aerobic exercise that is easy on the spine.

Spine Care (I and II). Glen Braatz, D.C. Minneapolis: Spine Care Publishers, 1962, 1976. Two booklets packed with information about exercise, posture, and lifting. Contact Spine Care Publishers, 3954 Wooddale Ave., Minneapolis, MN 55416.

Total Body Training. Richard H. Dominguez. New York: Warner Books, 1983. Includes exercises for the back recommended by chiropractors.

Index

Page numbers in *italics* refer to figures in the text.

About the Author

Nathaniel Altman graduated from the University of Wisconsin in 1971. He has authored more than a dozen books on vegetarianism, holistic health, Indian philosophy, and hand analysis including *Eating for Life*, *The Palmistry Workbook*, *The Nonviolent Revolution*, *Living With Asthma*, and *Lovelight: Unveiling the Mysteries of Sex and Romance* (with Julia Bondi). He lives and works in Brooklyn, New York.